# THE
# WHOLE-FOOD
# GUIDE *for*
# BREAST CANCER
# SURVIVORS

## A NUTRITIONAL
## APPROACH
## *to* PREVENTING
## RECURRENCE

EDWARD BAUMAN, MED, PHD
HELAYNE WALDMAN, MS, EDD

NEW HARBINGER PUBLICATIONS, INC.

Eating for Health and Vital Scoop are trademarks of Bauman College: Holistic Nutrition and Culinary Arts, a 501(c)(3) nonprofit educational institution

Distributed in Canada by Raincoast Books

Copyright © 2012 by Edward M. Bauman and Helayne L. Waldman
New Harbinger Publications, Inc.
5674 Shattuck Avenue
Oakland, CA 94609
www.newharbinger.com

Cover design by Amy Shoup
Acquired by Wendy Millstine
Edited by Nelda Street

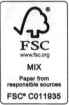

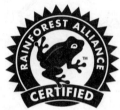

FSC
www.fsc.org
MIX
Paper from
responsible sources
FSC® C011935

Library of Congress Cataloging-in-Publication Data

Bauman, Edward M.
  The whole-food guide for breast cancer survivors : a nutritional approach to preventing recurrence / Edward M. Bauman and Helayne L. Waldman ; foreword by Donald Abrams.
     p. cm.
  Summary: "The Whole-Food Guide for Breast Cancer Survivors presents an integrative whole-foods nutrition and lifestyle plan for enhancing immunity and preventing cancer reoccurrence. The program highlights the foods, supplements, and natural remedies that can help people keep cancer from coming back"-- Provided by publisher.
  Includes bibliographical references and index.
  ISBN 978-1-57224-958-5 (pbk.) -- ISBN 978-1-57224-959-2 (pdf e-book)
  1. Breast--Cancer--Nutritional aspects. 2. Breast--Cancer--Prevention. 3. Diet therapy.
4. Self-care, Health. I. Waldman, Helayne L. II. Title.
  RC280.B8B382 2012
  616.99'449--dc23

                              2011044071

Printed in the United States of America

17      16      15

10      9      8      7      6

# DEDICATIONS

*This book is dedicated to my beloved mother, Jane Mann Bauman; to women grappling with breast cancer; and to oncologists. May the latter embrace whole-food nutrition to enhance treatment outcomes and create vibrant postcancer lives for their patients.*

—Ed Bauman

*This book is dedicated to my loving and inspiring father, Robert Waldman; my extraordinary Tanta Yetta; and my dear friend Kathleen Hogan—all taken by cancer too young. I know that writing this book is exactly what you would want me to do.*

—Helayne Waldman

# CONTENTS

# FOREWORD

Whereas most of us appreciate how tobacco use contributes to the development of avoidable malignancies, only 50 percent of us recognize that what we eat and avoid eating are equally important. Actually, the proportion of avoidable cancer deaths caused by diet is very close to that of those related to tobacco. Increasing awareness of this association between nutrition and malignant disease will likely be the main thrust of future health care reform, which will put more of an emphasis on prevention and wellness than our current disease management system does.

Diet is important not just for reducing risk, but also for helping patients live with, and beyond, cancer. The relationship between nutrition and cancer is an area of great concern to the integrative oncologist, whose main focus is not on the cancer per se but on the person living with the disease. In this context, we can say that cancer is like a weed. The surgeon, radiation oncologist, and medical oncologist are adept at dealing with this weed. The integrative oncologist then works with the entire garden, making the soil as inhospitable as possible to the growth and spread of this weed. And what better way to do so than to closely examine how people fertilize their gardens, by carefully reviewing what they eat?

In my integrative oncology practice, I spend most of my consultation hour discussing how best to fertilize the garden. I encourage patients to consume an organic, plant-based, antioxidant-rich, anti-inflammatory whole-food diet. What a joy to have *The Whole-Food Guide for Breast Cancer Survivors* to add to my list of recommended reading! Ed Bauman and Helayne Waldman have provided us with a practical and palatable recipe for adding both quality and quantity to the lives of the women and their families who access this vital information. Each chapter offers goals, steps to take, a to-do list, and a "Last Word" from a survivor, making the information easy to digest and assimilate. Excellent tables, including super recommendations on how to jazz up a salad, and an assortment of delicious, healthy recipes ensure that many readers will file this book in the kitchen for future reference. The thoughtful sample meal plan is just what people are always asking for to help apply the broad recommendations made by their nutrition-savvy care providers.

Although this whole-food guide targets the breast cancer survivor, its appeal is really universal. The information contained herein is just as valuable to men with prostate cancer, people with colorectal cancer, or anyone with any malignant diagnosis. Other than perhaps the specific references to hormone manipulation through diet and supplements, the advice to address deficiencies and excesses, to manage weight, to manage glucose and insulin levels, to enhance immunity, and to decrease inflammation are applicable to all patients, regardless of their cancer diagnosis. In fact, these recommendations are just as relevant for those aiming to reduce their risk of malignant disease (as well as heart disease and other degenerative diseases of aging) as they are for those seeking to thrive after treatment.

Two-thirds of Americans are now obese or overweight—a setup for increased disease burden and premature mortality. Clearly we have lost our sense of how to interact with food. This is not really the fault of the individual, as our political-industrial complex has done much to promote unhealthy eating habits. A cancer diagnosis is often a great motivator for behavior change. Breast cancer survivors who may not have been as conscious of healthful nutrition prior to diagnosis will find *The Whole-Food Guide for Breast Cancer Survivors* to be an invaluable resource in the ensuing chapters of their lives. Hopefully they will share the information with their families and friends—both with and without cancer—to promote health and well-being for all.

—Donald I. Abrams, MD
Integrative Oncology, UCSF Osher Center for Integrative Medicine
Chief of Hematology-Oncology, San Francisco General Hospital
Professor of Clinical Medicine, University of California, San Francisco
Past President, Society for Integrative Oncology

# ACKNOWLEDGMENTS

The idea for this book first started rumbling when Helayne attended the Evidence-Based Complementary and Alternative Cancer Therapies Conference, a breathtaking source of information and advocacy produced annually by Ann Fonfa of the Annie Appleseed Project. We would like to thank Ann for her vision and inspiration, and for empowering thousands of individuals to take charge of their health by understanding how to reduce the risk of cancer recurrence.

Of course, it takes a lot more to bring an idea to fruition, and for that, there are many others to thank. First, heartfelt thanks to our colleagues and other professionals who took the time to talk or consult with us and to review our ideas and material to ensure that the medical concepts were clear and correct. These generous souls include Donald Abrams, MD; Jeffrey Dach, MD; Connie Hernandez, ND; Robert Kane, DC; Bruce Ames, PhD; Joyce McCann, PhD; Chris Melitis, ND, NMD; David Brownstein, MD; Jonathan Wright, MD; Mary Ellen Chalmers, DMD; Sara Gottfried, MD; and Helayne's good and incredibly helpful friend, Michael Rosenbaum, MD. Additional thanks are due Cristiana Paul, MS, Nutrition Science; Carolyn Bernstein, NP; Jodi Friedlander, NC; Jason Miller, LAc; Judy Lane, NP; Rebecca Murray, NP; Mindy Toomay; Molly Colin; Lindsey Berkson, MS; Jeanne Wallace, PhD; Beth Gillespie, MS; Linda Lizotte, RD; chef extraordinaire Rebecca Katz, MS; and chef *fabuloso* Lizette Marx.

In addition, we would like to acknowledge Ralph Moss, PhD, whose writings on cancer have informed so many people, and whose books and website have been a wealth of information that has helped to shape and inform this book.

Several students from Bauman College volunteered to take on various assignments, for which we are most grateful. We send thanks to Gail Gummin, Maria Quintana, Debbie Miller, Tara Miller, Mia Rosingana, Leyla Bilge, and the supertalented Sela Seleska and Laura Halpin, for their valued contributions. Thanks also to Alana Kivowitz of UCSC.

Many thanks to Wendy Millstine and Jess O'Brien at New Harbinger Publications for their help, encouragement, and enthusiasm for this project. Thanks also to Nelda Street for her meticulous copyediting.

I would like to specifically acknowledge my mother, Jane Mann Bauman, who passed away from breast cancer thirty years ago. Her loss prompted me to make a lifelong commitment to helping women with this issue to receive both medical and complementary health care to improve their quality and duration of life.

I am grateful for the love and support of my wife, Chris Clay Bauman, my lifelong sweetheart and partner in health who created the Eating for Health graphic, and to my daughter, Jessica, who is an inspiring young woman and devoted daughter.

Thanks, too, to my colleagues and students at Bauman College and clients at Bauman Nutrition clinic, who are eating and living for health day in and day out, touching the lives of their friends, families, and community both near and far.

—Ed Bauman, MEd, PhD

Sometimes help comes in the form of "virtual angels," people whom you have never met but who, through the magic of cyberspace, have become friends, guides, and wonderful fountains of wisdom. D'Ann Smith has been one such remarkable angel, along with other cyberspace wisewomen: Marilyn Holasek Lloyd, Karla Jones, Sally Gould, and Carole Berlin.

It is impossible to put together a project of this scope and magnitude without the support of friends and family. Warmest gratitude to Susan Gordon, Margaret Wyles, Miriam Kook, Ken Schulman, Leah Shelleda, and Justin Isaacs for their invaluable feedback and support, with a special shout-out to Deanna Gould, Fran Glushakow Gould, and Jill Arnel, who went the extra mile to help make critical things happen.

Extraordinary thanks are due Mira Dessy, who started as an intern and has become a close friend and colleague, helping with every aspect of writing and editing this book.

Finally, thank you to Julie Preston for being the wonderful daughter, researcher, and editor that you are, and to my husband, Rob Kavet, without whom this book could not have been born.

—Helayne Waldman, MS, EdD

# INTRODUCTION

Few things are more devastating to a person's peace of mind than a cancer diagnosis. It brings up fears not only for our own health but also for the well-being of our families, friends, and loved ones. For this reason and because it takes the lives of thousands of Americans every day, cancer has been the subject of intense scrutiny for half a century and has been studied for more than one hundred years.

Scientists have come to the conclusion that cancer is a chronic disease of the genome that can appear in anyone at any time, triggered by genetic predisposition *and* a confluence of interactions with the environment. Yet not everyone with the breast cancer gene develops the disease. Whether a woman avoids developing breast cancer, genetics notwithstanding, has everything to do with a myriad of other factors, including exposure to environmental factors, diet, lifestyle, stress, and more.

Once a woman is diagnosed with breast cancer, an inevitable fear permeates her body and mind, and her friends and family are affected as well. Alarming questions emerge: *Why did this happen to me? Why now? How serious is this illness? What treatment will be suggested? What can I do to improve my chances of having a happy and healthy life after treatment? If this cancer goes away, how can I minimize the risk of recurrence?* Too often, some of these important questions go unanswered.

Despite doctors' best intentions and high level of skill at diagnosing and treating cancer, there is still a great deal that we don't know about this most frightening of diseases. Fortunately, there is a new movement within medicine that addresses the health of the whole person, not just the presence of cancer. This movement, *integrative oncology*, draws on traditional and contemporary natural health and wellness philosophies in addition to conventional cancer treatment modalities, resulting in a multifaceted approach to supporting the well-being of women with breast cancer.

Prominent among the wellness factors that a woman can proactively address every day of her life is nutrition. Good nutrition is the very foundation of cancer resistance, a vital, life-enhancing component of lifelong tissue growth as well as tissue damage, repair, and recovery. Emphasizing certain foods while avoiding others is a powerful self-care practice, and the healthy food choices presented in this book for that purpose are delicious and satisfying to boot.

For the woman whose life has been turned upside down by a cancer diagnosis and treatment, optimal nutrition is key. This book offers an Eating for Health approach, which supports a healthy liver; digestive, immune, and hormone balance; nutrient sufficiency; and positive genetic expression. We explain the mechanisms of cancer, provide evidence-based information on how to prevent or delay its onset or recurrence, and offer suggestions for supporting sustained recovery. Dr. Bernie Siegel, who, along with his wife, Bobbie, founded the Exceptional Cancer Patients (ECaP) center in New Haven, Connecticut, articulates the whole-person approach we share. In working with people who have cancer, he writes (quoted in Hughes and Hughes 2006):

> ...your actions depend on your attitude. If you listen to a doctor who tells you, "You have two months to live," you can go home and be dead in a week. You just turn off everything. But what if you got angry at the doctor and said, "Who are you to tell me when I'm going to die?" Then you might go home and start fighting for your life to prove the doctor wrong. What a difference! So that's why I began to learn from people who didn't die when they were supposed to. They all have stories to tell you. They were not denying their mortality, but they were using it to truly begin to

experience life and do what felt good before they died. However, once you're feeling good, it's a benefit to your body and the healing process, and this is why we have spontaneous remission. It's crazy to me that we don't study success. Somebody has an incurable disease but survives, but we don't rush to them and say, "How did you manage this?" We just say it's a miracle.

Our book aims to give women who are dealing with breast cancer instruction and support about risk and diagnosis, both before and after treatment. This information can enable integrative oncologists to share the care of cancer patients with nutrition consultants, natural chefs, and other healing arts and mental health professionals. We seek to create a network of health professionals who provide coordinated nutritional and personal support, elegantly blended with medical treatment.

# Nutrition Is Power

The Eating for Health approach to improving eating habits and food choices supports health and contributes to protecting healthy cells from becoming cancerous; it doesn't claim to be curative. If we assume that cancer is a genetic disorder, our focus is on which foods support cancer-protective gene expression versus which foods promote cancer proliferation. The research on this nutrition-based approach is still emerging, because foods have not been studied as exhaustively as botanical and, especially, pharmaceutical medicines.

Because few researchers have tested the healing power of diet alone for breast cancer, we see the role of food and nutrients as promoting health and peace of mind, and supporting life. Jeffrey Bland, a pioneering biochemist in the field of nutrigenomics, has stated (2010) that fresh, whole plant foods speak to our genes in a language they understand, encouraging them to function in a health-promoting way (more on this in chapter 3). It is logical to conclude that consuming foods that were grown in poor soil, and then overprocessed and blended with chemical additives, colors, and preservatives, is less conducive to health in general due to such foods' low nutrient content and tendency to arouse inflammation at a cellular level. We will explore this premise in detail in the chapters to come.

# Engaging the Whole Person in Healing

For healthy women, this book provides reliable nutritional information that can help you to stay cancer free. If you have had breast cancer, we explain how to use nutrition and lifestyle practices to minimize the chance of a recurrence.

Nutrition for the body comes from food; nutrition for the soul comes from hope, faith, and love. Combining optimal bodily nutrition from fresh, whole foods with soul nutrition from kindness and compassion communicates to our genes that we are committed to making the most of life. Whatever toxicity, trauma, or malnutrition may have contributed to the altered gene expression that we call cancer, these patterns may shift as we surround ourselves with love and good wishes while undergoing treatment. If indeed an ounce of prevention is worth a pound of cure, then our intention is to provide you with information, skills, and Eating for Health guidelines and recipes that you can use to foster vibrant health. May you live a long, full life knowing that the "C" word stands for many things besides cancer, including courage and commitment to change and growth.

## A MESSAGE FROM A SURVIVOR

To those facing diagnosis or recurrence, I'm delighted to welcome you to this book by Ed Bauman and Helayne Waldman. Being a breast cancer survivor myself and having worked with hundreds of breast cancer patients over the last fifteen years, I think I have a pretty good idea of what goes through someone's mind when she is dealing with a cancer diagnosis or is concerned about recurrence. You may first experience some panic and fear, but I hope learning and enlightenment will quickly follow. Everyone who has been through this experience is overwhelmed at first.

If you are currently in a place of panic or fear, it will pass, and you will be ready to move on to educating yourself. The most exciting part about learning about breast cancer is that there is so much to learn, and there are so many aspects of this disease we can take into our own hands to improve our own outcomes. This book provides a road map to these steps.

A lot of information is contained herein, so do not expect to read this book as quickly as you might read a book-club selection. Go through this book at a pace that's comfortable for you; you may sometimes have to put down the book and pick it up the next day where you left off. The book isn't going anywhere, nor is the information. Take your time with the material, reading and rereading the parts that pertain especially to you.

The speakers who come to my conference each year and the authors of this book talk a lot about *biochemical individuality*, which means that some risk factors discussed here may pertain to you and others may not. The point of individualized care and self-care is to recognize and understand your individual differences and to work with them first and foremost. So concentrate on the chapters that call your name. There is no right or wrong way; there is your way. Making informed decisions is what works best.

It may help to take notes along the way on issues you may want to discuss with your practitioner. I encourage you to discuss what you read with your practitioner to get his or her perspective and to share yours (you are *so* important to the decision-making process). The "To Do" list at the end of each chapter is your guide to taking action. Refer to each list as many times as you need to help put your personal plan in motion. The material will become second nature to you before you know it. Refer to the appendixes for all sorts of backup information, such as pantry lists, recipes, and suggested testing. This is not a one-time read; rather, it is a resource that you can refer to again and again. Remember that the "Last Word" sections are all from women who have successfully taken the same journey as you—women like me.

Finally, I suggest using this book not as a stopping place, but as a jumping-off place. Find areas that are relevant, and follow up with your own research. There's nothing more empowering than walking into your practitioner's office with a wallop of data, and an open and curious mind. Best of luck on your journey from one who has been there and back!

—Ann Fonfa
Breast cancer survivor,
founder and director of the Annie Appleseed Project

# Chapter 1

# Reviewing Traditional Risk Factors

*I'm not afraid of storms, for I'm learning how to sail my ship.*

—Louisa May Alcott

CHAPTER GOAL: Review well-known risk factors

Learning how to sail your ship is what this book is all about. Amid the troubled waters of a breast cancer diagnosis or the risk of one, there is great hope, because every year, we learn more about sailing our ships.

In this first chapter, we'll start by reviewing risk factors that have been well documented over the past several decades. Except where otherwise indicated, all of the data contained in this chapter were provided by the National Cancer Institute (NCI) (2011) and the American Cancer Society (ACS) (2011b). Some of these risk factors cannot be changed. In subsequent chapters, however, we'll look at more recently discovered risk factors and their profound implications. These new discoveries are especially exciting, because they are *modifiable risk factors*, meaning that your *own* dietary and lifestyle choices can have a profound impact on your ability to modify your risk level. And that's great news to anyone with concerns about breast cancer.

## Traditional Risk Factors

This generation of women in the United States faces a greater lifetime risk of breast cancer than any previous one, with rates having tripled during the past forty years, according to holistic nurse educator and clinical nutritionist Susan Luck (2010). In fact, the NCI (2010) estimates that 12.15 percent (one in seven) of women born in 2009 will be diagnosed with breast cancer at some time in their lives. And if you've already had breast cancer, you're undoubtedly concerned about your risk of recurrence.

### Gender

Being female is, by far, the most substantial risk factor. According to the ACS, the incidence of breast cancer is about 100 times higher in women than in men. The explanation for this difference is not the number of breast cells per se, but rather the contact female breast cells have with the growth-stimulating effects of female hormones.

Race also plays a role in breast cancer. According to the ACS, Caucasian women have a higher incidence of breast cancer, although more African American women die from it. Asian Americans, Hispanics, and Native Americans appear to have a lower risk of both incidence and death from breast cancer.

## Age

Your risk of developing any illness increases with age. It is now estimated that one in eight *invasive* breast cancers (cancers that invade surrounding areas) are found in women who are younger than age forty-five, and unfortunately risk rises steeply with age. Two out of three cases of breast cancer in women aged fifty-five and older are considered invasive.

## Weight

Prior to menopause, your ovaries produce most of your estrogen, while fat tissue produces only a small amount. After menopause, the ovaries shut down production, and most of your estrogen comes from the adrenal glands and fat tissue. Having more fat increases your estrogen levels, which can raise your chance of developing breast cancer, and it appears that having more abdominal fat may increase your risk. What's more, women who are overweight have higher levels of circulating insulin. Insulin, being a growth factor, is an independent risk for breast cancer, a topic we'll expand on in chapter 6.

## Lack of Physical Activity

Lack of physical activity not only leads to weight gain but also may be another factor that increases your risk of developing breast cancer. The Women's Health Initiative (WHI) (McTiernan et al. 2003) found that "as little as 1.25 to 2.5 hours per week of brisk walking reduced a woman's risk by 18 percent." The ACS recommends forty-five to sixty minutes of physical activity, five or more days per week.

# Genetic Factors

Fortunately, only 5 to 10 percent of breast cancers result directly from mutations due to inherited genetic defects. The much-publicized BRCA-1 and BRCA-2 genes are examples of these defective genes. If you inherit a mutated copy of either of these genes, your risk of developing breast cancer escalates to as high as 80 percent. What's more, when breast cancer strikes women with these genes, it happens at a younger age and tends to show up, more often than not, in both breasts (*bilateral presentation*). Jewish woman of Eastern European descent have the highest incidence of this genetic pattern, although it can occur in any race or ethnic group. Other alterations in genes, such as p53, ATM, CHK2, and CDH1, increase breast cancer risk as well. Modern technology allows us to identify these aberrant genes through specialized genetic testing (see appendix B). This testing is not routinely provided to women with concerns about breast cancer risk, although a doctor can order it at the patient's or a family member's request at any age.

# Hormonal Factors

Cumulative lifetime exposure to estrogen is considered a risk factor for breast cancer, so early puberty (before age twelve), and late menopause (after age fifty-five) each add to your risk. Other hormonal factors include the timing of pregnancy, breastfeeding, weight, exposure to oral contraceptives, use of hormone replacement therapies, and use of the synthetic estrogen *diethylstilbestrol* (DES).

## EARLY PUBERTY

The rising rate of obesity in our youth may be a contributing factor to early puberty since body fat can produce the sex hormones that lead to glandular development. The notion that environmental chemicals that mimic estrogen may contribute to an earlier onset of puberty has been suggested but remains unproven (Grady 2010).

## PREGNANCY STATUS

While early pregnancy is known to offer protection, a benefit of natural hormonal changes, both late pregnancies (after age thirty-five) and no pregnancy at all confer a statistically higher incidence of breast cancer.

## NO BREASTFEEDING

Known to provide many health benefits for the baby, breastfeeding also appears to offer protective benefits to the mother by helping to reduce her risk of developing breast cancer, especially when infants breastfeed up to one to one-and-a-half years of age.

## ORAL CONTRACEPTIVE USE

Several studies have uncovered a link between the long-term use of birth control pills and breast disease later in life. A noteworthy NCI-sponsored study published in 2003 (Althuis et al.) reported that using oral contraceptives generated a higher risk of breast cancer, especially in younger women. This risk was more pronounced in women who had used oral contraceptives within the past five years, whereas the risk diminished over a longer period (ibid.).

## HORMONE REPLACEMENT THERAPY

After years of recommending postmenopausal hormone replacement therapy (HRT) to millions of women, the medical establishment reversed course after the publication of the Women's Health Initiative Study in 2002 (Rossouw et al.), which reported that five years of combined HRT (pharmaceutical estradiol and progestin) was associated with a 26 percent increase in risk of invasive breast cancer in postmenopausal women.

## DIETHYLSTILBESTROL

Developed in the late 1930s, diethylstilbestrol (DES) is a synthetic estrogen that was administered to pregnant women to help prevent or lower the risk of miscarriage. Women who took DES and women whose mothers took it may have a higher risk of developing breast cancer. The ACS (2010a) provides information about the link between DES and breast cancer (see the references).

# Confirmed Environmental Exposures

Environmental factors are increasingly recognized as an important part of the risk of breast cancer. The biggest environmental risks, ones that you can, to some extent, control, are smoking cigarettes and working at night.

## SMOKING CIGARETTES

Although smoking is traditionally associated with lung cancer, we've learned from a number of recent studies that the risk of breast cancer is also strongly associated with smoking and secondhand-smoke exposure. The risk of breast cancer increases by 50 percent among women who have smoked for forty years or longer, compared to nonsmokers (Cui, Miller, and Rohan 2006).

Smoking is a clear and present risk factor for breast cancer. Although quitting can be an arduous task, the rewards are huge, and many organizations, including the American Cancer Society, can provide help (see appendix B).

## WORKING NIGHTS

While not as controllable as smoking cigarettes, working at night is an environmental factor. The ACS indicates that women who work night shifts, such as nurses and flight attendants, may have a change in melatonin levels (a hormone produced by exposure to light). This change is believed to be a factor that increases the risk of developing breast cancer.

# Keep in Mind

Despite the multitude of risk factors discussed here and elsewhere, it's empowering to remember that most people do *not* get cancer in their lifetimes and that most women who *do* get breast cancer survive the experience. In the following chapters, we'll look at all of the ways available to you to lower your risk and claim your rightful power to more confidently sail your ship.

## Last Word

*For years, cancer was just a word to me. Now it's a journey, filled with challenge, yes, but also the joy of learning.*

—H. Levy, breast cancer survivor

# CHAPTER 2

# EMERGING RISK FACTORS

*The terrain is everything.*

—Louis Pasteur

CHAPTER GOAL: Learn about emerging risk factors for breast cancer

In mid-nineteenth-century France, a vigorous war of ideas raged in the upper echelons of the scientific community. On one hand, Louis Pasteur was developing his germ theory of disease, and on the other, Claude Bernard was focused on the *milieu interieur,* or the internal environment of the host. Bernard felt that the nourishment of the body, its ability to get rid of toxins and wastes, and the strength of its immune system provided the foundation for successfully confronting both acute and chronic disease. Although Pasteur and others fought long and hard for the supremacy of the microbe theory of disease, Pasteur experienced a dramatic turnaround late in life and, on his deathbed, is said to have uttered, "Bernard was right. The microbe is nothing. The terrain is everything."

We wholeheartedly agree that healthy "terrain" is the foundation for a healthy body that can mount a strong defense against cancer. In this chapter, we'll cover the basics of emerging risk factors for breast cancer, the ones that deal with the internal terrain as Bernard or Pasteur might envision it today. These factors include dietary and nutritional influences, toxic exposures, and the health and equilibrium of the body's own internal systems, such as the hormonal, digestive, and immune systems. We consider these risk factors to be so important that we've devoted entire chapters to many of them later in the book. Others we'll just touch on briefly in this chapter.

# The Standard American Diet: Your Number One Risk Factor

The *standard American diet* (SAD), sometimes also referred to as the *Western dietary pattern,* consists of a high intake of red meat, sugar, trans fats, high-fructose corn syrup, artificial sweeteners, and refined grains.

This dietary pattern also includes a low intake of colorful, whole-food fruits and vegetables.

## The High Cost of Cheap Food

The health of the majority of Americans is getting worse as you read this. In the Time magazine article "Getting Real about the High Price of Cheap Food," Bryan Walsh (2009) writes, "Unless Americans radically rethink the way they grow and consume food, they face a future of... higher health costs." Why? Food experts, such as Michael Pollan, warn us that the quality of our food supply has been on a slow decline for many decades; that is, our food has become more toxic and less nutritious. In fact, much of what we eat is not actually food at all but what we like to call "UFOs," or "unidentified food objects." Just look at the label on a typical packaged food from a supermarket shelf. Try to pronounce most of the ingredients, and you'll see exactly what we mean. It's no surprise that we're witnessing an unprecedented rise in obesity, blood-sugar imbalances, autoimmune diseases, and cancer in our population (ACS 2010b).

The crux of the matter is this: fast food and packaged foods, as documented by Eric Schlosser in *Fast Food Nation* (2001) and Carol Simontacchi in *Crazy Makers* (2000), are made from the least-expensive ingredients possible and loaded with chemicals, damaged fats, artificial ingredients, and flavor enhancers. Fast foods *are* stimulating but *they are not* nourishing. Many experts, including researchers from the American Institute for Cancer Research (AICR) (2007), believe that for the twelve most common cancers, about 35 percent of cases in the United States are preventable through maintaining a healthy diet and healthy weight, and being physically active. So eating a diet aimed at risk reduction is probably the most important step you can take to lower your chances of dancing with this most unpleasant disease.

**Sick animals make for unhealthy food.** While consuming malnourished, pesticide-laden plants can lead people to appear sickly and malnourished, those same substandard crops, combined with excessive amounts of hormones and antibiotics, lead to sickness in animals. Factory-farmed animals are fed a steady diet of genetically modified (GM) corn and soy, with the intent of making the cattle gain weight quickly. What's more, a typical fast-food or school-lunch burger is not made from a single piece of beef, but from "meat" from a variety of sources, such as trimmings and scraps of fatty wastes that are left on the slaughterhouse floor after the animals have been butchered.

The same basic practices are also applied to raising chicken and fish. Simple common sense tells us that feeding GM soy and corn pellets to algae-loving salmon, or sawdust, hormones, antibiotics, and cardboard to insect-loving chickens, will produce sickly, malnourished animals, whose meat then contains the drugs, pesticides, and other toxins the animal consumed. Indeed you are what the animal on your dinner plate ate.

**Got rBST?** Studies over the past decade have pointed clearly to the fact that consuming cattle that were fed artificial growth hormones has led to increased rates of breast cancer, early puberty, and obesity in the United States (Bohlooly-Y et al. 2005). Monsanto first began selling recombinant bovine growth hormone (rBGH), also known as rBST (recombinant bovine somatotropin), in 1994. The hormone, designed to force cows to produce more milk, has been banned in Europe, Canada, Japan, Australia, and New Zealand due to safety concerns. Nevertheless, in the United States, Monsanto has insisted that its genetically modified growth hormone is safe. Many experts say otherwise. A key area of concern is the startling rise in human blood levels of a growth hormone known as insulin-like growth factor (IGF-1). As Dr. Samuel Epstein (1996), noted toxicologist, explains, consumption of animals that were fed growth hormones leads to excessive levels of IGF-1, a close relative of insulin, in humans.

Researcher Susan Hankinson first sounded the alarm on IGF-1 in 1998, when she and her colleagues reported that among seventy-six premenopausal women, those with IGF-1 blood concentrations in the highest third had almost three times higher risk of breast cancer than those with levels in the lowest third. And among premenopausal women younger than age fifty, the risk of breast cancer for those with the highest levels of IGF-1 was approximately *seven* times higher than for women with the lowest levels. "The up-to-sevenfold increase suggests that the relation between IGF-1 and risk of breast cancer may be greater than that of other established breast cancer risk factors, with the exception of a strong family history of breast cancer or a high-density mammographic profile," warned Hankinson and her colleagues.

Given the research, we consider it prudent to strictly moderate your intake of commercial animal products to help keep this risk factor under control. Since the USDA does not require labeling of milk containing rBST as of this writing, it is safe to assume that if your milk is not labeled organic or doesn't clearly state the *absence* of rBST, the cows that produced it were indeed treated with the hormone. The good news is that you can avoid this risk by choosing milk that is labeled "organic" or "rBST free."

## Sugar and Cancer: A Sweet Relationship?

You may already know that simple sugars and carbohydrates cause an almost immediate rise in blood glucose levels. The problem with this scenario is that cancer cells have a voracious appetite for sugar. Dr. Otto Warburg first discovered the connection in 1924, when his research revealed that cancer cells generate energy in a way that differs from normal cells, utilizing a process called *glycolysis*, a discovery for which he later won the Nobel Prize. He contended that this process was so dependent on glucose that he dubbed tumors "obligate sugar metabolizers": "Cancer, above all other diseases, has countless secondary causes. But, even for cancer, there is only one prime cause. Summarized in a few words, the prime cause of cancer is the replacement of the respiration of oxygen in normal body cells by a fermentation of sugar" (Warburg 1966). Warburg observed—and that observation has not been challenged in almost a century of subsequent research—that not only does consuming sugars and simple carbs rapidly raise blood glucose, but also the fast, abrupt nature of this increase triggers a healthy pancreas to respond by overproducing insulin in order to bring the levels down to a normal range as quickly as possible. This initially healthy response, however, can lead to very unhealthy consequences. Insulin and its close relative IGF-1 are powerful cellular growth promoters (Hadsell and Bonnette 2000). In other words, these hormones have the job of sending "grow" messages to your tissues.

The connection among blood glucose, insulin, and breast cancer has been documented for decades. For example, a 1985 mouse study (Santisteban et al.) indicated that higher blood glucose levels resulted in shorter survival times in mice with breast cancer, with the response being "dose dependent." In other words, the higher the blood glucose levels, the poorer the outcomes.

What's critical to understand is that simple carbohydrates (white bread, rice, pasta, pastries, and so on) convert to simple sugar within moments of your chewing them. Complex carbohydrates, those with intact fiber and germ, on the other hand, release their glucose more slowly and more healthfully into the bloodstream. We'll discuss more on sugar, insulin, and cancer in chapter 6.

## Time for an Oil Change?

Fats and oils have an intimate relationship with cancer, because they either promote or inhibit inflammation, a topic that we will discuss in detail in chapter 8. The nature of fats and oils changed dramatically about fifty years ago, when processed foods started coming into their own as a mainstay of the American diet. During those years, food manufacturers started looking for a way to preserve the shelf life of processed foods as well as home and industrial cooking oils and fats. Very quickly, genuine fats became factory fats; that is, they were replaced with hydrogenated trans fats, a new, lab-created fake fat that was completely foreign to the human body.

So what happens when you actually eat this stuff? Because trans fats are similar in chemical composition to real fats, your body believes that they are real, and uses them in all the places where real fats are designed to go—especially the all-important cell membrane. In the words of diet guru Sally Fallon (2001), your cells actually become partially hydrogenated! Why is this a problem? Because all nutrients and waste products must pass through this vital cellular gatekeeper (the cell membrane), we cannot afford to have membranes that are rigid and hard, inhibiting the smooth exchange of nutrients and waste products. We'll talk a great deal more about fats that are friends and fats that are foes in chapters 3 and 8.

## America's Other Drinking Problem

In the United States, we're told that our water is among the purest in the world, but a closer look reveals a startlingly different story. Vital to health and to life, clean water is the only liquid the body actually needs, and nothing can replace it. Opinions vary as to how much we need each day (48 to 64 ounces, by most accounts), but need it we do, whether it comes from our food, our tap, or bottles. In 2009 the Environmental Working Group (EWG) disclosed that more than 260 contaminants had been detected in tens of thousands of samples of tap water, many of them petrochemicals and their by-products. What's more, over half of the contaminants were unregulated. Of these unregulated toxins, the EWG concluded that 53 are linked to cancer, 41 to reproductive toxicity, 36 to developmental toxicity, and 16 to immune-system damage. For others, no health information seems to exist at all.

Based on these troubling findings, the pollution of our water seems to be one more possible contributor to the ever-growing cancer epidemic in our country. We'll provide tips for locating and filling up on healthy drinking water in chapter 4.

# Nutritional Deficiencies and Efficiencies: When Food Isn't Enough

A well-nourished body boasts a thriving community of healthy cells, and healthy cells are more resistant to oxidative stress and DNA damage, two factors that increase the chances of their becoming cancerous. Well-nourished cells are also capable of interacting with one another more effectively, making sure that all cells work together as a coordinated community. What's more, when they are damaged or worn out, healthy cells die in an orderly process known as *apoptosis*.

As much as we advocate the use of whole, nutrient-dense food as a foundation for wellness and cancer prevention, there are many instances when the purest, freshest proteins, fats, carbohydrates, and *phytonutrients* (protective chemicals made by plants) from food simply aren't enough. We can lay the blame on depleted soil producing less-nutritious crop yields, on toxins in our environment, on endocrine-disrupting chemicals that throw our hormones out of balance, or on digestive issues that prevent us from absorbing and using the nutrients available in the food we eat. Indeed, all of these factors share some of the responsibility, because they all lead to a state of nutrient depletion, which, in turn, leads to a state of diminished health. That's where targeted nutritional supplementation comes in.

Vitamin D, iodine, and selenium are just three nutrients that have been shown to play a dominant role in cellular and immune health. Copper and iron, in excess, on the other hand, have demonstrated the capacity to *hasten* cancer's progression. We'll take a closer look at the relationship of specific nutrients to the risk of breast cancer occurrence or recurrence in chapter 5.

## Immune Capability

One way of reducing your risk of breast cancer occurrence or recurrence is to have a healthy immune system, one that recognizes unhealthy cells and destroys them. Cancer, however, is exceedingly cunning in its ability to evade immune surveillance, secreting chemicals designed to camouflage it and confuse our cellular defenders. Think of it as a Trojan horse that cloaks itself in a devious array of disguises to throw your immune system off-track. When your army of T cells, phagocytes, and natural killer (NK) cells—the specific cells that fight cancer—is well nourished and well rested, your immune system has a better chance of mounting a swift and strong response to cancerous cells before they can multiply and become dangerous.

One of the greatest risks to immune health, and one that we *can* completely control, again, involves the intake of sugar and refined carbohydrates. Excess sugar depresses immunity, as was shown as far back as the 1970s (Sanchez et al. 1973), when subjects ingesting 75 to 100 grams of a sugar solution (about 20 teaspoons of sugar, or the amount in two average 12-ounce sodas) showed a dramatic drop in neutrophil count, a measure of white blood cell activity. This plunge happened within fifteen minutes of eating a high-glycemic meal, and although the immune suppression was most noticeable two hours after ingestion, the effect was still evident five hours after eating. We'll delve more into this and other factors affecting immune health in chapter 7.

## Inflammation Stokes the Fire

A fire can spread quickly and devastatingly, or slowly, making it easier for firefighters to subdue. Inflammation is the fire in the growth and spread of cancer. In a healthy body, inflammation represents a protective response to an emergency, such as invasion by a bacterium, virus, or parasite. Inflammation is a time-tested process that initiates the body's innate healing process, a lifesaving response to wounds and infections that might not heal without it. An inflammatory state can become chronic, however, which is when it causes problems.

The same inflammatory chemicals that are used to heal wounds can promote cancer growth. One way that this happens is when white blood cells rush to the site of an injury, initiating the development of new blood vessels in a process known as *angiogenesis*. What's more, inflammation seems to play a variety of roles in all phases of cancer: its initiation, promotion, and invasion (Sgambato and Cittadini 2010).

Fortunately, we are well aware of several natural anti-inflammatory foods and nutrients. *Quercetin*, a bioflavonoid phytonutrient found in apples, onions, and tea; curcumin; ginger; and omega-3 fatty acids are among the best. Likewise, sunlight, which allows the body to make vitamin D, is a natural antioxidant and is anti-inflammatory.

Identifying and eliminating food sensitivities is another key to alleviating undue inflammation. By discovering your own particular food sensitivities, you can avoid foods that are provocative to your system. This is one key to taming the inflammation beast, but we'll discuss several others in chapter 8.

## The Breast Cancer–Iodine Connection

According to Dr. David Brownstein (2008), author of *Iodine: Why You Need It, Why You Can't Live without It*, iodine is one of the most essential nutrients for breast health. In fact, decades of work have been painstakingly undertaken to confirm this protective role. It is believed that iodine does its work through modulation of gene expression and estrogen containment, while remaining intimately involved in the process of cell division and replication, and apoptosis, the process of normal cell death (ibid.).

From epidemiological studies, we learn that iodine deficiency is linked to a higher rate of goiter and breast cancer, undoubtedly because iodine exerts the lion's share of its effect on both thyroid and breast tissue. Conversely, high levels of iodine intake are associated with reduced goiter and breast cancer rates (ibid.). Japan, for instance, has the highest dietary intake of iodine (approximately 13 milligrams per day), and the lowest rates of goiter and breast cancer (ibid.). Interestingly, when Japanese women move to the United States and consume the same amount of iodine as American women, their breast cancer rates increase. Dr. Brownstein (personal communication) has tested more than four thousand patients in his practice, and his results have been remarkably consistent: over 95 percent of his patients are iodine deficient. How can this be, when our saltshakers are brimming with iodized salt? Perhaps it's because Americans also consume three other chemicals in large amounts that compete with iodine for absorption: fluoride, chlorine, and bromide. In chapter 5 we'll talk more about these iodine-disrupting chemicals and what you can do to make sure that you have enough iodine to confer the maximum degree of breast cancer protection.

## Gut and Liver Health

Several theories of cancer development emphasize the concept of "total load," or the cumulative amount of toxins that your body is challenged to neutralize on a day-to-day basis. When this load gets too heavy to carry, the liver, our primary detoxification organ, can no longer keep up with the job of clearing out waste products. As the wastes continue to build, they recirculate, and they damage, first, our cells as a whole and then the DNA *inside* our cells. By supporting a healthy liver and digestive tract, we help to move toxins through and out of the body, minimizing toxic overload and excessive DNA damage. A healthy liver is also critical in detoxifying human estrogens and foreign estrogen compounds, called *xenoestrogens*, which can initiate and accelerate breast cancer growth (Aschengrau, Rogers, and Ozonoff 2003). We call this good cellular housekeeping.

Cruciferous vegetables, beets, curcumin (from the spice turmeric), and carotenoids, found in carrots, tomatoes, oranges, and many other fruits and vegetables, are particularly good at supporting the liver in breaking down toxic additives, pesticides, hormones, and other chemicals that can threaten our health.

The liver is an organ with awesome executive responsibility; treat it well, and it will return the favor. More on this in chapter 9.

## Handling Hormones

All women manufacture a variety of estrogens throughout their lifetimes. Before menopause, the ovaries produce these estrogens, and after menopause, the adrenal glands and adipose (fat) tissue make them, albeit in smaller amounts. Women who are overweight have more adipose tissue, so they produce more estrogen. What's more, these estrogens do not distribute themselves evenly around the body. In menopausal and postmenopausal women, excessive levels of estradiol, the most dominant estrogen, commonly accumulate in breast tissue, creating an additional risk of developing estrogen-dependent tumors.

The real crux of the matter, however, is not how much estrogen we have, but how we *metabolize* the estrogens that we produce. An imbalance of estrogens in the body can actually set the stage for cancer development and proliferation, particularly in postmenopausal women. Depending on your diet, your liver's detoxification abilities, and the quantity and quality of healthy flora in your gut, you can safely metabolize and excrete excess estrogen in the form of the healthful estrogen metabolite known as *2-hydroxyestrone*, or you can recycle a more toxic, rogue estrogen metabolite known as *16-alpha-hydroxyestrone* (Eliassen et al. 2008). We'll look into these distinctions in chapter 10, where we'll draw on the wisdom of Dr. Jonathan Wright, a leading expert on female hormones.

# CAT Scans and Other Sources of Radiation

Two research studies were recently published that disclosed that CAT scans deliver a great deal more radiation than previously believed (Redberg 2009). One NCI study, in fact, which came to the attention of the public in a 2009 *USA Today* article (Szabo), found that patients experiencing such scans may be exposed to up to four times more radiation than previously estimated; in fact, one study concluded that one CAT scan could expose a patient to as much radiation as 74 mammograms or 442 chest X-rays (Smith-Bindman et al. 2009).

It's also worth noting that, although controversial at this time, some experts believe that yearly mammography screening may give insufficient benefit to certain groups of women to justify the additional radiation exposure. These concerns spurred the U.S. Preventive Services Task Force (USPSTF) to recommend sweeping changes in its breast cancer screening guidelines in 2009, in a controversial move that advocated for less-frequent mammograms.

We believe that appropriate screening can be a lifesaving procedure. Which form of diagnostic screening you use is a critically important and highly personal decision that you and your doctor must weigh carefully against all known risks of such procedures. While we don't actively support one form of screening over another (in fact, they are often most powerful in combination), we do support the importance of educating yourself about the risks and benefits of each procedure you choose to undertake, and of discussing the risk-benefit ratio with your health care practitioner.

# Nurturing Your Terrain

As we pointed out at the beginning of this chapter, the internal terrain that you foster within your body is one of the most critical factors that will influence the course of either benign or cancerous breast disease. And now, we'll turn our attention to the specifics of managing that terrain.

### Last Word

*Of course cancer doesn't grow in a vacuum. You can either encourage it or discourage it by what you put in your mouth, in your lungs, and on your body every day. That's the first thing I learned.*

—Stefanie R., breast cancer survivor

# CHAPTER 3

# EATING FOR HEALTH FOUNDATIONAL PLAN

*Would you really rather have broccoli or a sticky bun talk to your genes?*

—Robert Rountree, MD, May 2010, National Association of Nutrition Professionals conference

> CHAPTER GOAL: Understand the foundational plan for healthy eating—Eating for Health

Is it nature or nurture that determines our susceptibility to cancer? One of the most exciting concepts in modern nutrition, *nutrigenomics*, teaches us that it isn't one or the other, but a combination of both. Nutrigenomics looks at how foods can trigger genetic changes for good or ill. Through the efforts of nutrigenomic scientists, there is growing evidence that good dietary choices can help prevent the onset of cancer and may even help cure it.

You might believe that your genetic code is what it is and that it determines many things about your health status over your lifetime. This is partly true, but a variety of influences can alter your DNA at any time, and even in the absence of any genetic tendency, breast cancer can result. If your genes do predispose you to develop breast cancer, take heart: not all people with a predisposition will develop cancer. Whether or not the disease actually occurs depends on a host of complex interactions between your genes and your overall "ecosystem," your body's basic "terrain."

The food you eat; the water you drink; the air you breathe; all the chemicals you encounter in cosmetics, medicines, and cleaning products— everything that your body is subjected to on a day-to-day basis—affect the functioning of your bodily systems, your vital organs, and your very genes, providing stimuli that either can bring a particular genetic trait to full expression or subdue its impact.

In fact, according to the National Institutes of Health (NIH) (2007), only about 5 to 10 percent of all breast cancers are hereditary. The vast majority of breast cancers are attributable to other causes, which are currently under investigation by countless research scientists. At least three theories continue to be heavily researched: that chronic inflammation can lead to cancer, that an excess of oxidation is to blame, and that a compromised immune system can contribute to development of the disease.

Because diet can have a profound effect in all three of these areas, it makes good sense to regularly consume antioxidant-rich, anti-inflammatory, and immune-stimulating foods, while avoiding foods that are more likely to cause disease. That's what our Eating for Health plan is all about.

Research shows that health and well-being are best served when beneficial fats, complex carbohydrates, and lean proteins are consumed in appropriate proportion day in and day out, along with a wide variety of phytonutrients, health-boosting compounds abundant in fruits, vegetables, and other plant foods that provide protection against cancer and other diseases.

The Eating for Health plan focuses on emphasizing just such foods in your diet, providing a blueprint for avoiding cancer triggers while consuming plenty of cancer preventers. If cancer is discovered in your body, dietary choices can contribute to slower progression of the disease, better tolerance of treatments like chemotherapy and radiation, and longer survival times (Dolecek et al. 2010).

As the pace of modern life increases along with our exposure to toxins in air, food, and water, the need for a wide variety of protective foods and nutrients also increases. Fortunately, the rewards of eating seasonal, chemical-free, nutrient-rich, organic foods include not just disease prevention and healing, but also increased energy, more-balanced moods, and better-managed weight—as well as wonderful flavors, textures, and aromas at the table.

The modern food industry favors an economy of scale, which is less about health and nutrition and more about long shelf life and profit. Fortunately, healthy alternatives are burgeoning, and organic foods, farmers markets, and hormone-free, pasture-fed animal products are now easily accessible in many areas of the country. If they are not available locally, you can even order fresh and frozen organic food delivered to your door from online markets, such as Planet Organics (www.planetorganics.com).

Eating for Health (E4H) offers a nondogmatic, flexible approach to meeting your body's needs for optimal nutrient quality, quantity, and diversity. Ed first designed the E4H model in 1991 as an alternative to the USDA food pyramid, which reflected the biases of the meat, dairy, cereal, soda, and snack-food industries. In addition to mapping health-promoting food and beverage choices, E4H promotes the idea of ensuring that you have clean air, pure water, and an active lifestyle that includes stress reduction, healthy sleeping patterns, and regular social support.

# Eating for Health and Breast Cancer

Eating for Health is the *beginning* of your breast cancer nutritional recovery strategy, not the end. Our aim is that you start with the recommendations in this chapter, then use the ensuing chapters to customize the program based on your own unique needs and biochemistry. That's how it works best.

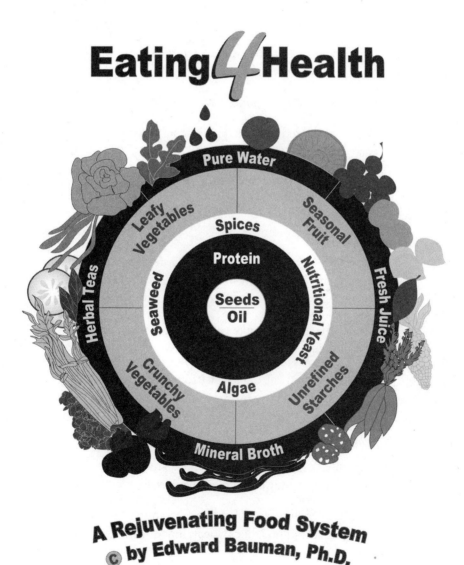

Eating 4 Health

Pure Water
Leafy Vegetables
Seasonal Fruit
Herbal Teas
Spices
Protein
Nutritional Yeast
Fresh Juice
Seaweed
Seeds Oil
Algae
Crunchy Vegetables
Unrefined Starches
Mineral Broth

A Rejuvenating Food System © by Edward Bauman, Ph.D.

# Eating for Health Guidelines

Eating for Health is based on science and sustainability. Here are some guidelines to help you embrace this new way of relating to food. You may want to check off the ones you already follow, and star the ones you intend to add to your daily routine:

_____ Grow your own salad greens and herbs, and if you have a large yard, cultivate fresh fruit or nut trees, or berry vines.

_____ Drink plenty of filtered water each day, about one-half cup (4 ounces) every hour.

_____ Read labels and avoid foods with artificial ingredients.

_____ Avoid eating refined and artificial sugars, especially in pastries and confections.

_____ Eat more vegetables; learn to love legumes!

_____ Consume breakfast before 10:00 a.m. and include a serving of good-quality protein.

_____ Have protein at three-to-four-hour intervals during the day to curb sugar cravings and stabilize blood sugar and insulin production.

_____ Minimize caffeine intake to 50 milligrams a day or less for women, and twice that for men.

_____ Choose monounsaturated fat (from olives, avocados, almonds, macadamia nuts) or virgin coconut oil over fat from commercial meat and dairy or polyunsaturated oils (soy, corn, sunflower).

_____ Decrease consumption of glutenous grains (wheat, rye, and barley), which may cause digestive disturbance.

_____ Increase consumption of gluten-free grains (rice, organic corn, millet, quinoa, buckwheat, amaranth).

_____ Have two or more servings of colorful vegetables per meal for optimal pH (acid-alkaline) balance. Overacidity causes inflammation and depletes the body of calcium, magnesium, sodium, and potassium (Frassetto et al. 2000).

_____ Add "booster" foods, such as algae, sea vegetables, nutritional yeast, and culinary spices, to your diet to increase trace minerals, which aid healthy metabolism, detoxification, and antioxidant activity.

_____ Eat slowly, with blessings and gratitude.

# Macronutrient Basics

When we talk about macronutrients, we're referring to complex carbohydrates, protein, fat, and fiber. We'll look briefly at each one from an Eating for Health perspective.

## Protein

The Eating for Health model advises eating _unadulterated_ protein from fresh sources. By unadulterated, we mean that the precious amino acids comprising the protein have not been stripped out, burned, overheated, extruded, overprocessed, or tampered with in any significant way. As you might expect, that leaves out such items as commercial (nonorganic) dairy, grilled meats, and any factory-farmed animal products.

_Protein_ literally means "of prime importance." No wonder; protein is essential for building and repairing tissue, for producing enzymes and hormones, and for regulating fluid balance in the body. To ensure maximum assimilation, we suggest having several small portions of protein throughout the day, approximately 12 to 20 grams per serving, depending on your age, activity level, weight, and health status. Excellent choices are wild, fatty fish; organic, free-range animal meats and eggs; fermented, unprocessed soy products (miso, natto, and tempeh); legumes; whole grains; nuts; seeds; and algae.

**About Protein and cancer.** While small amounts of grass-fed beef can be very healthy, it is important to avoid overconsuming red meat, because it lowers the body's pH. Cancer tends to thrive in an acidic environment (pH of 6.8 or lower) and is stymied in an alkaline environment (pH greater than 7) (Gatenby et al. 2007). To track where you are on the acid-alkaline scale, keep a stock of pH strips on hand, available at any drugstore, to check your saliva before eating or drinking anything in the morning. If your salivary pH is lower than 6.8, you can take action by adding more fresh fruits and vegetables and herbal teas to your diet.

**Soy protein.** Eating soy can be a good alternative to meat. For example, one cup of tempeh contains about 24 grams of digestible protein, as well as soluble fiber, zinc, B vitamins, iron, calcium, and magnesium. What's more, unadulterated soy protein shows great promise in the prevention and management of cancer, as shown by several large epidemiological studies, such as the Shanghai Women's Health Study, in which soy food intake was shown to decrease the risk of premenopausal breast cancer (Shu et al. 2009). Soy products appear to inhibit breast cancer by decreasing levels of circulating estrogens through the action of special chemicals known as *genistein* and *daidzein*.

There are potential problems with soy protein, however. You'll want to consider the following issues:

- *Digestibility:* Many people find it difficult to digest soy, and are reminded of this in no uncertain terms when they experience gas, bloating, and indigestion. Should these symptoms occur, try cutting back on portion sizes or taking a digestive enzyme at the beginning of your meal. Your digestive system may have an easier time with tempeh, miso, or natto, all fermented soy foods enjoyed regularly in Asian countries, especially Japan. The process of fermentation increases digestibility of all foods, *including* soy. Fermenting soy also inhibits the activity of *goitrogens*, natural thyroid-blocking agents found in unfermented soy.

- *Genetic modification:* Recently, a great deal of concern has been raised about the long-term safety of genetically engineered (GE) soy, which now constitutes approximately 80 percent of all soybeans grown (Center for Food Safety 2011). Developed by Monsanto, GE soy is grown from a special seed that is resistant to Monsanto's Roundup, a potent and controversial herbicide. This resistance allows much heavier doses of pesticide to be used on the crop, doses many experts believe to be toxic. And many questions remain about the safety of GE crops overall. For this reason, we very strongly recommend eating only organic soy foods. Be aware that *soy protein isolate*, a highly processed form of soy protein, often genetically modified, is used as a filler and additive in hundreds of food products. If you become a conscientious label reader, you'll be able to quickly recognize which products contain GE soy.

- *Soy controversies.* Soy is one of those foods that you either love or hate. In recent years, soy has been touted as a wonder food by the likes of physician Andrew Weil, while it has been vilified by others, such as nutritionist Kaayla Daniel (2005). Is soy indeed either healthy or hazardous for breast cancer survivors?

  We believe that if soy is organic and close to its original form, it can be a healthy addition to the diet. A cup of warm miso broth, some edamame, or a tempeh stir-fry can provide high-quality protein in addition to isoflavones, which act as weak estrogens, helping to guard estrogen receptors from more potent, aggressive estrogens.

  The Japanese typically eat soy from an early age, which may be one key to their lower rates of breast cancer. In April 2008, researchers (Iwasaki et al.) used blood and urine samples to measure isoflavone levels in almost 25,000 Japanese women. Those who had the highest levels of genistein (a soy isoflavone) had the lowest rates of breast cancer.

  Other studies provide mixed and often confusing results, depending on the age group of the women tested, the length of time soy products have been eaten, what other treatments are being used, and other variables.

  Using an Eating for Health approach can help sort through the confusing data. E4H supports the use of whole, organic soy, eaten in moderation, just as it supports the consumption of all whole foods. We do not recommend that you use soy as your sole source of protein, and we definitely advise against the use of all "fake" soy products, such as soy bacon, soy chicken, soy meatballs, and other "foods" created from soy-based, textured vegetable protein. These are not whole foods and, as such, would fall outside the scope of an E4H lifestyle.

We also suggest that you stay away from soy isoflavones as a supplement, because some experts have postulated that too much concentrated soy could fuel the growth of an existing tumor (ACS 2010c). There is also concern that soy might counteract the protective effects of tamoxifen (Ju et al. 2002). If you have trouble digesting soy or have thyroid issues, it is best to avoid it altogether.

## Carbohydrates

Carbohydrates are the water-soluble starches and sugars in food that provide energy to the body, modulated by the hormone insulin. Complex carbohydrates, such as unadulterated whole grains; root vegetables and tubers, like yams and turnips; and an abundance of fresh, organic, and seasonal vegetables and fruits provide the fiber, B-complex vitamins, and minerals the body needs to support the health of the gastrointestinal (GI) system and to satisfy our appetites.

According to advocates of low-carbohydrate diets, as Americans' intake of carbohydrates has increased, so has the incidence of obesity, cancer, and heart disease. While this is true, most low-carb guidelines fail to clarify the difference between complex and simple, refined carbohydrates. Complex carbohydrates provide generous amounts of B vitamins, zinc, magnesium, chromium, vitamin E, and fiber. Simple, refined carbohydrates have these nutrients removed. Sadly, Americans have been sold the myth that synthetic vitamins, when added to refined carbs, are as good as or better than the original, naturally occurring nutrients that were removed. The Eating for Health plan recommends only consuming complex carbohydrates in their whole, unprocessed form.

## Fabulous Fiber

The E4H model advises eating high-fiber foods, such as whole grains, vegetables, and legumes, to fully benefit from both insoluble and soluble (sometimes called "viscous" or "gooey") fiber. Both types of fiber are plentiful in plant foods, because they are the structural part of the plant itself. A diet high in both kinds of fiber speeds transit time through the intestine and fosters regular elimination, helping to flush toxins, including excess estrogen, from the body. Some good sources of insoluble fiber are organic whole grains; nuts and seeds; the bran of various grains; fibrous vegetables, such as celery, green beans, and leafy greens; and the skins of fruits and vegetables. Important sources of soluble fiber include oats and oat bran, dried beans and peas, barley, flaxseeds, nuts, and psyllium husk.

**Bad news for cancer: fiber stabilizes blood sugar.** The positive effect of fiber on blood sugar and insulin is important in preventing all types of cancer, including breast cancer. Both insoluble and soluble fiber (but especially soluble) help to normalize blood glucose levels by slowing the rate at which sugars are absorbed into the bloodstream. This keeps blood sugar and insulin levels lower, which denies a growing tumor both the sugar and insulin it needs to thrive. We'll discuss this in detail in chapter 6.

### Fats

Although seeds and oils take up little space in the E4H model, they are in the bull's-eye, a very prominent position, because fat is crucial to our survival and is our greatest source of energy. Healthy fats build and maintain healthy cells, insulate tissues, protect our organs, and make up more than half of the gray matter in our brains. Healthy fats also help us absorb fat-soluble nutrients, such as vitamins A, D, E, and K; maintain the health of our skin, hair, and arteries; and stabilize blood sugar levels. Without enough healthy fat in our diets, we would become ill, indeed.

## Phenomenal Phytonutrients: Fruits, Vegetables, Herbs, and Spices

Plant foods contain literally thousands of beneficial compounds, including macronutrients, *micronutrients* (vitamins and minerals, the subject of chapter 5), and phytonutrients (*phyto* means "plant"), protective chemical compounds that occur naturally in plants. Biochemist and Nobel laureate Albert Szent-Gyorgyi first discovered the tremendous power of a family of phytonutrients called *flavonoids* in 1936.

Thousands more phytonutrients have been discovered since 1936, most of which are now known to be faithful defenders against all types of illness. Phytonutrients abound in the fruits of some plants, in the leaves or stems of others, and in the skin or white pith of still others. These phenomenal phytos act in a synergistic way with other nutrients to regulate critical bodily functions, such as those controlled by the liver and the immune, nervous, and endocrine systems. Choosing an artificial-chemical–free E4H plan takes full advantage of these phytonutrients in the form of fruits, vegetables, and "booster" foods, such as herbs, spices, and seaweeds, which are critical pieces in the puzzle of maintaining and restoring good health.

## PLANT FOOD: YOUR FIRST LINE OF DEFENSE

We want to clearly emphasize that food is your best line of defense against breast cancer and its spread. That said, due to biochemical individuality and a history of insufficient micronutrient and phytonutrient intake, targeted supplementation with specialized nutrients may provide valuable backup support. However, we are aware that some folks believe they are getting an insurance policy by washing down their fast food with a chaser of vitamins. This is not a winning strategy! In fact, a report from the Department of Food Science, Cornell University, asserts that "the additive and synergistic effects of phytochemicals in fruits and vegetables are responsible for…potent antioxidant and anticancer activities and that the benefit of a diet rich in fruits and vegetables is attributed to the complex mixture of phytochemicals present in whole foods" (Liu 2004).

With that, let's look at some of our favorite cancer-fighting foods.

---

## TO DO: Top-15 Hit Parade of Cancer-Protective Foods

Foods work on multiple body systems to nourish, cleanse, and heal. An E4H diet provides six to twelve servings a day of fresh, whole fruits and vegetables. Each of the following plant foods contains as many as one hundred cancer-protective phytonutrients. Some of these phytonutrients have been consistently associated with elements of cancer protection and healing in population-based epidemiological studies; others show great promise in laboratory and animal research but are still awaiting confirmation in human research. If you haven't already tried these foods or made them a part of your weekly routine, you'll want to add them to your to-do list right away!

| Food | Proposed Active Constituents | Proposed Activity* |
|---|---|---|
| Apple | Phenolic compounds | Inhibit cancer cell proliferation, reduce inflammation (Lapidot, Walker, and Kanner 2002) |
| Bitter melon | Eleostearic acid | Induces cell-cycle arrest and apoptosis (Kobori et al. 2008) |
| Berries | Flavonols, hydroxycinnamic acids, anthocyanins, and phenolics | Inhibit cell proliferation, lower all inflammatory markers (Yi et al. 2005) |
| Broccoli | Sulforaphane, indole-3-carbinol | Inhibit breast-cancer stem-cell activity, inhibit cancer-cell motility, enhance detoxification (Gamet-Payrastre et al. 2000) |
| Celery | Apigenin, luteolin | Inhibit aromatase activity (Way, Kao, and Lin 2004) |
| Fatty fish (wild) | Omega-3 fatty acids | Anti-inflammatory, downregulate cancer-promoting PcG gene (Dimri et al. 2010) |
| Flax | Lignans, omega-3 fatty acids | Reduce inflammation, downregulate HER-2 expression (Thompson et al. 2005) |
| Garlic | Diallyl disulfide | Reduces cell adhesion and invasion (Lei et al. 2008) |

| Food | Proposed Active Constituents | Proposed Activity* |
|---|---|---|
| Green tea | Epigallocatechin-3-gallate (EGCG) | Inhibits a number of tumor-cell proliferation and survival pathways (Thangapazham et al. 2007) |
| Lemon | D-limonene, citrus pectin, auraptene | Reduce cancer cell adhesion, downregulate IGF-1 and other growth factors (Poulose et al. 2007) |
| Mushrooms | Polysaccharides | Enhance immune system, facilitate cancer-cell cytotoxicity (in vitro) (Martin and Brophy 2010) |
| Pomegranate | Ellagitannins | Facilitate antiproliferative and anti-aromatase activity (Adams et al. 2010) |
| Seaweed | Fucoidan, iodine | Detoxify, promote apoptosis (Yamasaki-Miyamoto et al. 2009) |
| Turmeric | Curcuminoids | Inhibit cell proliferation and invasion, lower inflammation (Bachmeier et al. 2008) |
| Whey protein | Immunoglobulins, lactoferrin | Inhibit proliferation of mammary epithelial cells in vitro and in vivo (Liao, Du, and Lönnerdal 2010) |

* The studies cited here are representative of the many hundreds of studies undertaken to examine the relationship between food and breast-cancer risk and development. Although these and other experimental results are very promising, it is important to remember that results in a test tube (in vitro) do not always translate into results in a human body. Animal (in vivo) studies, on the other hand, can offer significantly improved predictive value, because there are more similarities than differences between humans and laboratory animals.

## EATING FOR HEALTH SAMPLE MEAL PLAN

| | Day 1 | Day 2 | Day 3 | Day 4 | Day 5 |
|---|---|---|---|---|---|
| **Breakfast** | Protein-rich smoothie ½ to 1 C oatmeal with almonds 1 C green tea 1 C water with lemon | 2 poached eggs ½ C kale 1 tbsp. flaxseeds ½ C blueberries 1 C green tea 1 C water | Protein-rich smoothie ½ to 1 C oatmeal with almonds 1 C green tea 1 C water with lemon | 1 C seasonal fruit ¼ C walnuts ½ C goat yogurt 1 C green tea 1 C water with lemon | Protein-rich smoothie ½ to 1 C oatmeal with almonds 1 C green tea 1 C water with lemon |
| **Snack** | 1 small apple 2 tbsp. Brazil nuts 1 C coconut water | 8 baby carrots ¼ C edamame beans 1 C water with lemon | ½ C hummus 1 C raw veggies 1 C herbal tea | 2 to 3 tbsp. almonds 1 orange or tangerine 8 oz. water 1 C green tea | 1 nori sheet 1 oz. goat cheese 10 celery sticks 1 C water |
| **Lunch** | 2 tofu soft tacos with salsa, lettuce, tomato, cilantro ½ avocado 1 C herbal tea 1 C water | 3 oz. baked chicken 1 C mixed green salad ½ C quinoa | 1 to 2 C rice pasta with shrimp and veggies 1 C water 1 C lemonade | ½ C brown rice ½ C steamed cauliflower ¼ C seaweed salad | 1½ C Spicy Winter Squash and Red Pepper Bisque (p. 182) ½ C quinoa Red Cabbage Salad (p. 186) 1 tbsp. olive oil with lemon 1 C water |
| **Snack** | ½ C hummus 1 C raw veggies 1 C herbal tea 1 C water with lemon | 1 scoop green powder (such as Vital Scoop or Biopharma Scientific NanoGreens) 8 oz. water 1 C green tea | 2 tbsp. pumpkin seeds 1 small apple 1 C miso soup 1 C water | 1 C popcorn 1 tbsp. nutritional yeast ½ tsp. tamari 1 tsp. olive oil 1 C herbal tea | 1 small apple 2 tbsp. almonds 1 herbal tea |
| **Dinner** | 3 oz. grilled salmon 1 C Swiss chard ½ C brown rice 1 tsp. olive oil Side green salad 1 C water with lemon | 2 Lentil and Millet Burgers (p. 179) 1 C broccoli 1 tablespoon olive oil 1 C water with lemon 1 C ginger tea | 3 oz. baked halibut 1 C Brussels sprouts ½ C brown rice 1 tbsp. flaxseed oil 1 C herbal tea 1 C water with lemon | 1½ C lentil soup with chicken ½ C quinoa ½ C beets 1 small salad 1 C water | 3 oz. salmon ½ C kale ½ C maitake mushrooms 1 small yam 1 tbsp. olive oil 1 C water with lemon |

# Final Thoughts: A Call to Consciousness

Eating for Health is more than a dietary program. It's a way of thinking, feeling, and living that emphasizes a return to more traditional, whole foods, eaten mindfully and with the intention to feed and nourish the body while communicating a gentle, peaceful message to your genes and DNA. It's a return to nature for nourishment.

## Last Word

*For me, my cancer diagnosis was a call to action, an invitation to examine my daily habits and make changes for the better. I learned that true healing happens one bite at a time, one sip at a time, one breath at a time, with an attitude of gratitude for the chance to share love and live with purpose. By embracing the principles of Eating for Health, I feel that I have learned how to live well by eating well.*

—Debbie M., breast cancer survivor

# CHAPTER 4

# AVOIDABLE EXPOSURES

*Then a strange blight crept over the area, and everything began to change.... There was a strange stillness.... The few birds seen anywhere were moribund; they trembled violently and could not fly. It was a spring without voices. On the mornings that had once throbbed with the dawn chorus of scores of bird voices, there was now no sound; only silence lay over the fields and woods and marsh.*

—Rachel Carson, from *Silent Spring*, September 1962

> CHAPTER GOAL: Learn how to limit your exposure to toxins to a manageable level

With the publication of *Silent Spring*, Rachel Carson inspired a generation. For the first time in human history, millions of people learned that the indiscriminate use of pesticides threatened both their health and that of the planet. Through scrupulous study and observation, Carson ascertained that in nature, where all species are interconnected, chemicals aimed only at insects were soon ingested by other animals and passed up the food chain. "As few as eleven large earthworms can transfer a lethal dose of DDT to a robin," Carson wrote (1962, 108). "And eleven worms form a small part of a day's rations to a bird that eats ten to twelve earthworms in as many minutes." Carson's work spawned an engaged and active environmental movement, and although it can boast many successes (such as the banning of the pesticide DDT), it has also faced a number of escalating challenges in the ensuing decades, as more and more hastily tested or untested chemicals have been released into the environment.

Pollutants and chemical contaminants can activate cancer in a variety of ways. In this chapter we'll take a look at some of them.

# The President's Cancer Panel

Although Rachel Carson lit the spark, it wasn't until 2010 that a firestorm was finally ignited with the publication of the President's Cancer Panel report (Leffall and Kripke), *Reducing Environmental Cancer Risk: What We Can Do Now*. The 200-plus-page report was the first of its kind to concentrate on environmental connections to cancer and, for that reason, was widely praised by environmental organizations and health professionals alike.

The report asserts that "the true burden of environmentally induced cancers has been grossly underestimated" (ibid., iii), which would seem to advocate for precise steps to reduce the public's pervasive exposure to cancer-causing agents, or *carcinogens*. Particularly prominent in the report was a critique of bisphenol A (BPA), used in plastic bottles and can linings, as well as the toxic elements radon, formaldehyde, and benzene. "A precautionary, prevention-oriented approach should replace current reactionary approaches to environmental contaminants in which human harm must be proven before action is taken to reduce or eliminate exposure," the report warns. "This approach should be the cornerstone of a new national cancer prevention strategy that emphasizes primary prevention" (ibid., xi).

As advocates of proactive risk reduction, we concur. With that in mind, this chapter will examine some of those chemicals with demonstrated ties to breast cancer, and what you can do to minimize your exposure to them.

# Personal Care Products

Although women put all sorts of lotions, creams, conditioners, antiperspirants, and makeup on their faces and bodies daily, these products are not necessarily safe. The cosmetics industry remains one of the most unregulated in the United States, with its products falling outside the jurisdiction of the Food and Drug Administration (FDA) *and* the U. S. Department of Agriculture (USDA). This means scarce oversight, burdening the consumer with the job of evaluating the safety of each product purchased.

Among the more common chemicals we find in these mysterious mixtures known as "personal care products" are lead, mercury, and phthalates, the latter of which is a plastic additive used in not just cosmetics but also in children's toys, plastic bottles, and many other household items.

Dr. Samuel Epstein (2009), author of *Toxic Beauty: How Cosmetics and Personal Care Products Endanger Your Health…and What You Can Do about It* and chairman of the Cancer Prevention Coalition (preventcancer.com), has done an extraordinary job of categorizing and documenting the hazardous ingredients in unregulated personal care products, referred to often as "cosmeceuticals." Many of these products contain what Epstein calls "hidden carcinogens," ingredients that activate or discharge powerful toxins, such as formaldehyde and nitrosamines, and go by names like methenamine, polyoxymethylene, DEA, TEA, and PEG. Other products are tainted with carcinogens like ethylene oxide, dioxane, and acrylamide (www.ewg.org/skindeep/).

43

# More Than Skin Deep

Even more disturbing is the recent popularization of products that use *nanoparticles*, microscopic bits of the previously mentioned ingredients, which penetrate the skin effortlessly and, due to their microscopic size, can also invade blood vessels, traveling throughout the bloodstream to other organs. In May 2006, Friends of the Earth, a global network of grassroots groups, published the report (Miller) "Nanoparticles, Sunscreens, and Cosmetics: Small Ingredients, Big Risks," which advocates that these suspect personal-care products should be taken off the market to protect public health.

# The Cost of Teenage Beauty

We are particularly concerned about the widespread use of multiple personal care products by teenaged girls and young women. When the Environmental Working Group (EWG) conducted a study of teenaged girls (ages fourteen to nineteen) in 2008 (Sutton), an astonishing 100 percent of them showed evidence of both methyl paraben and propylparaben in their blood and urine. It is especially disconcerting that such a chemical onslaught can happen during the critical developmental window of the teen years; therefore we urge all women, especially mothers of teenaged girls, to consult the EWG website (ewg.org) for suggestions and more information on personal care products. A few of these suggestions follow:

- Use fewer commercial products and simpler, more natural ones.

- Don't rely on claims like "dermatologist tested" or "natural." Become an avid label reader.

- Avoid "antiaging" creams, many of which use potentially dangerous nanoparticles.

- In particular, steer clear of products and ingredients that have been linked to cancer and hormone disruption, such as:

    - Antiperspirants containing mineral oil, aluminum compounds, fragrances, and silica (we suggest avoiding all antiperspirants)

- Dark, permanent hair dyes
- Fragrances and dyes
- Nail polish and removers
- Parabens
- Triclosan and triclocarban

- Opt for lemon, avocado, tea tree oil, aloe gel, or some combination of them as beneficial ingredients.

- Buy products from trusted vendors that use only nonhazardous ingredients. Check out the website of The Campaign for Safe Cosmetics (safecosmetics.org) for suggestions.

- As a good starting place for your research, use EWG's Skin Deep Cosmetics Database (www.ewg.org/skindeep).

From Helayne's experience, we can also recommend the following:

- Essential oils make wonderful perfume, without the risk. Experiment with lavender, patchouli, and other scents that appeal to you.

- Coconut oil is a luxurious skin moisturizer and makeup remover.

- Baking soda is an effective facial scrub and underarm deodorant. It also makes a good toothpaste!

- Pure glycerin soap works as well as any, especially for sensitive skin.

- Xylitol (a natural sweetener) and water make an effective antibacterial mouthwash.

- Mashed avocado makes a delicious facial treatment that nourishes the skin.

- Applying pulped red hibiscus flowers to your hair is great for softness and shine (rinse out after thirty minutes). If you are using dried flowers instead of fresh, add water to make a paste.

- Jojoba oil is an easily absorbed, soothing oil from the seed of the jojoba plant, known for its affordability and low incidence of allergic reactions. Reported to be rich in skin-nourishing micronutrients, such as vitamin E, zinc, and silicon, this oil is easily absorbed into the skin and leaves no messy residue.

# Troubled Waters

We have a problem: a drinking problem. Turn on your kitchen water faucet or purchase a leading brand of bottled water and what do you get? It all looks and tastes like clear, clean water, but you might be surprised to learn that what we see is not what we get. In fact, in 2003 the Natural Resources Defense Council (NRDC) reported that although a vast number of contaminants affect the country's water supplies, some occur with far greater frequency than the rest and are directly related to cancer:

- Toxic chemicals include arsenic, radioactive radon, the herbicide atrazine, and perchlorate from rocket fuel, along with other suspected carcinogens, such as the gasoline additive methyl tertiary butyl ether (MTBE) and perchloroethylene (PCE). PCE transmitted from the plastic linings of asbestos-cement water-distribution pipes slightly to moderately increases breast cancer risk (Aschengrau, Rogers, and Ozonoff 2003).

- While disinfection of water supplies has dramatically cut down on waterborne illnesses, decaying organic matter reacts with chlorine to produce a host of other undesirable chemicals, known primarily as trihalomethanes (THMs). Chloroform is one of the better-known THMs, all of which are carcinogenic even in small amounts, as noted two decades ago when the *American Journal of Public Health* published a report (Morris et al.) showing a 15 to 35 percent increase in certain types of cancer among people who drink chlorinated water.

- Acrylamide, a carcinogenic compound that is formed when carbohydrates are fried at high temperatures (think French fries, doughnuts, potato chips), is also a by-product of the disinfection process, where it plays a part in the removal of solids from source water (EPA 2005).

In 2009 the EWG disclosed that more than 260 contaminants had been detected in tap water samples, 53 of which were linked to cancer.

## Hitting the Bottle

In response to fears about tap water, we have turned to bottled water as our reprieve for contaminated water and as a convenient alternative to commercial beverage choices when we're away from home. But, as lax as the EPA has been about tap water, the federal regulations for bottled water are even looser concerning testing for microbial agents and mandated disinfection. What's more, when plastic water bottles get hot, compounds in the plastic (also known as *phthalates*) can leach into the water, creating a high dose of xenoestrogens (chemical estrogenic compounds).

## Tips for Safe Water

Don't worry; there are ways to make your drinking water safe and healthy. But to make an informed decision about the right water-treatment system for your home, you must know what is in your water.

You can start by calling your water supplier or health department and requesting copies of water quality reports. Find out how often the water is tested, what it is tested for, and whether any violations are on file. You can also find out about any known hazards, such as lead, that might get into the water between the treatment plant and your tap. The best filter is inadequate if it doesn't filter out the right substances. Filters that have been independently certified to remove particular contaminants are your best bets. NSF International (nsf.org) is probably the best-known organization for setting standards for water filters and certifying them.

Carbon filters, reverse osmosis filters, and water ionizers all have different benefits and disadvantages, and range widely in price. When you are ready to buy, it is best to consult with an independent professional who can help you decide what's right for you based on an assessment of your tap water, your health concerns, and your budget. You might also consider buying a showerhead filter, because many contaminants can be absorbed through the skin or inhaled in steam.

For a compendium of excellent information on both municipal water and well water, you can also consult the consumer information about water on the Environmental Protection Agency (EPA) website: water.epa .gov/drink/info/.

# Pesticides

Pesticides are used to kill crop-destroying insects, while herbicides are used to kill undesirable plants, which means that both are intentionally toxic. Although pesticide use has doubled every ten years since 1945, the pesticides themselves are less successful at eradicating pests today than they were then (Crinnion 2000). Thus, more and more of them are needed to achieve their goal.

Ongoing research continues to detect new hazards in pesticides, often at doses once declared nontoxic by their manufacturers and the government. *DDT* (dichloro-diphenyl-trichloroethane), a useful but hazardous pesticide with far-reaching health effects, was proclaimed to be safe until its use was prohibited in 1972. DDT and other organochlorine pesticides are still so pervasive that they have secured the unglamorous designation *persistent organic pollutants* (POPs), meaning that they persist for decades in soil, air, and water. All animals, including humans, that eat, drink, and breathe these pollutants store them in their fat.

Connections between breast cancer and pesticide exposure have been acknowledged for decades, although in this century the research has dramatically accelerated, in part because the Centers for Disease Control (CDC) and other organizations have embraced the practice of *biomonitoring*. According to the CDC (2009), this technology allows scientists to test the concentration of contaminants in people's blood and urine in a more direct way than ever before. More than a decade ago, some pioneering Danish researchers used biomonitoring to verify that the risk of breast cancer was notably higher in women with high levels of the pesticide dieldrin (Høyer et al. 1998). Dozens of other studies have been published with similar findings. In fact, in June 2007, the journal *Cancer* devoted an entire supplemental issue to "Environmental Factors in Breast Cancer," stating (Brody et al.): "Laboratory research has shown that numerous environmental pollutants cause mammary gland tumors in animals; are hormonally active, specifically mimicking estrogen, which is a breast cancer risk factor; or affect susceptibility of the mammary gland to carcinogenesis." While some pesticides cause harm by impairing the immune system, others promote higher levels of dangerous estrogens (Muñoz-de-Toro et al. 2006). Still other pesticides may influence the degree of tumor aggressiveness (Demers et al 2000).

How relevant are animal studies to human health? According to the World Health Organization (WHO) (2006), "All known human carcinogens that have been studied adequately for carcinogenicity in experimental animals have produced positive results in one or more animal species." What's more, approximately 99 percent of mouse genes are identical to those found in humans (Mouse Genome Sequencing Consortium 2002). Accordingly, we pay close attention to animal studies.

## Guidelines for Avoiding Pesticide Exposure

The easiest way to avoid pesticides is to avoid pesticide-laden produce. The EWG (www.ewg.org/foodnews/) has identified twelve fruits and vegetables that it dubs "the dirty dozen," those doused with the highest levels of pesticide (as of 2011): apples, celery, blueberries, collard greens, grapes (imported), kale, nectarines (imported), peaches, potatoes, spinach, strawberries, and sweet bell peppers.

You will find most organic produce labeled as such at the store. If you're not sure, just look at the sticker on the product; all organic produce is labeled with a number beginning with 9. Wash all fruits and vegetables carefully, even organic ones, to remove dirt and traces of pesticide residue.

# Plastics

Plastics are ever present in our lives. Phthalates, the compounds that give plastics their flexibility, are involved in virtually every step of the food preparation, delivery, and storage chain. Commercial food is commonly processed using plastic equipment. Plus, it is packed and distributed in plastic-lined boxes and cans, most of which contain the chemical bisphenol A (BPA), an alleged endocrine disruptor and carcinogen. At home, many people deposit and then reheat leftovers in plastic containers that can transfer small particles of plastic into the food. The salt, fat, and acid found in many foods make matters worse by facilitating the transfer.

Phthalates are also contained in air fresheners, carpeting, cars, cleaners, computers, flea collars, floors, furniture, insect repellants, medical devices, nail polish, paints, perfume, PVC water pipes, rainwear, shampoo, shoes, shower curtains, shrink-wrap, teething rings, toys, varnishes, and many other consumer products (Berkson 2000). They are even used in pharmaceuticals to help enable timed-release dosing.

The association between phthalates and breast cancer has been hotly debated for over two decades. Plastic industry lobbyists (SPI 2009) claim that people's exposure to single-product compounds is well below toxic-exposure limits and causes no problems. Health experts and environmentalists (Takahashi and Oishi 2000) counter, however, that although exposure to one type of plastic may be below toxic thresholds, none of us is exposed to only *one* type of plastic. Europeans are taking no chances. Phthalates have been prohibited in cosmetics in Europe for decades (EU Council Directive 1976). The European Union widened its ban on phthalates in 2005 (EU Council Directive), issuing a directive against this highly suspect compound in children's toys and all oral child-care products.

## BPA: The New Bad Kid on the Block

BPA is a xenoestrogen; that is, it is thought to mimic the effects of estrogen in the body. You'll find it mainly in polycarbonate plastic bottles and the linings of food and beverage cans. It also finds its way into rivers, house dust, and just about anywhere official tests have been run. Like phthalates, it winds up in the food with which it comes into contact, particularly when that food is prepared at high temperatures.

In a 2007 survey, the EWG examined common sources of BPA in foods and the degree of exposure in people, and reported that:

- Over half of ninety-seven cans tested contained BPA. Chicken soup, canned ravioli, and infant formula had the highest levels of BPA of all products tested. Of four hundred people tested, BPA was detected in over 95 percent of them.

- For one in ten cans of all food tested and one in three cans of infant formula, enough BPA was found in a single serving to expose a person to more than two hundred times the government's designated safe level of BPA exposure for industrial chemicals.

The FDA does not offer oversight of BPA levels found in food, despite the fact that more than one hundred peer-reviewed studies have found BPA to be noxious even at low doses.

## POSSIBLE CONNECTION TO BREAST CANCER

BPA is apparently connected to breast cancer, although the risk seems to be more conclusive in infants whose mothers had high exposure during pregnancy. One group of animal researchers found that fetal exposure to low doses of bisphenol A "resulted in long-lasting effects in the mouse mammary gland that were manifested during adult life" (Murray et al. 2007).

The authors of *Our Stolen Future: Are We Threatening Our Fertility, Intelligence, and Survival?*, a book that examines environmental impacts on health, believe, as do other experts, that exposure of human fetuses to BPA also results in prominent changes in later breast development (Colborn, Dumanoski, and Peterson Myers 1996).

## GUIDELINES FOR AVOIDING BPA EXPOSURE

Are there precautions you can take at *your* stage of life? Of course. Clearly, if you are of childbearing age, it's critical to avoid contact with BPAs as much as possible. For the rest of us, lowering our body's burden of this toxic compound can only add to our well-being.

We consulted the EWG and the NIEHS (National Institute of Environmental Health Sciences) for their recommendations, which we include among ours:

- Minimize consumption of canned foods. EWG tests have found that BPA transmits from the liner of the can into the food inside the can.

- Avoid eating or drinking from polycarbonate plastics, used in products such as plastic baby bottles, sippy cups, and water bottles; food storage containers; and plastic eating utensils. It's easy to check for the type of plastic on the bottom of bottles; polycarbonate bottles, for example, are usually labeled with the number 7. Look for bottles and other containers made from glass, stainless steel, or nonclear plastic (which does not contain BPA). Note that certain metal water bottles are lined with a plastic coating that contains BPA. Look for stainless-steel bottles that are not lined with plastic (EWG 2007).

- Do not microwave food in polycarbonate plastic containers (NIEHS 2010).

- Do not drink from plastic bottles that have been sitting in a hot vehicle or that you suspect have been stored in a hot environment or previously frozen.

- Avoid handling credit card receipts, as they are coated with a thin layer of BPA (EWG 2010).

# Trust Your Eyes and Nose

Many other common consumer items are potentially harmful to our health and vitality, from secondhand smoke, household cleaning products, air fresheners, diesel fuel, house paints, building materials, furniture, flame retardants (PDBEs), and dioxins to leather goods, dental sealants, glue, dyes, art supplies, dry-cleaning compounds, and many more. Trust your eyes and nose to tell you what may be hazardous: if it makes your eyes tear up or your nose run, if it smells artificially strong, if it doesn't look or smell right, then it probably *isn't* right.

# Total Body Burden

Although pesticides, plastics, and pollutants can already be quite trouble-some as single agents, the reality of our environment is that they seldom appear alone. The concept of *total body burden*, sometimes referred to as *total load*, takes into account the collective effect of all the toxins to which we've been exposed. And since we have all been exposed, the question is not whether we've been exposed or even how much, but what can we do about it? In the book *Hormone Deception: How Everyday Foods and Products Are Disrupting Your Hormones—and How to Protect Yourself and Your Family*, D. Lindsey Berkson (2000) did a groundbreaking job of alerting us to our options for reducing our exposures. Refer to her book and use sug-gestions from the EWG as your guide. Of course, a nutrient-dense, Eating for Health diet goes a long way, too, in helping you lower your total load!

## To Do

While the scope and range of toxins in our environment can indeed be frightful, we suggest caution, not panic. By following the commonsense suggestions in this chapter, you are taking a big step toward creating a safer environment for yourself and your family, while lowering your risk of breast cancer and all other cancers. Here are some final to-dos, based on the work of both Berkson (ibid.) and the EWG (ewg.org/bodyburden /consumerproducts):

- Instead of Teflon cookware, use stainless steel (or cast iron if iron levels are not too high).

- Stay away from super-strength cleaners. Try nontoxic cleaning products like baking soda, borax, and vinegar. (Helayne has had great success with white vinegar.)

- Be sure to turn on the exhaust fan over your gas stove when you are cooking.

- Avoid stain repellents.

- Be mindful of breathing gasoline fumes from gas-powered lawn and garden tools.

- Wash all new clothes before wearing them and avoid traditional dry cleaning.

- Steer clear of commercial air fresheners and toilet deodorants. Instead, try baking soda to absorb odors.

- Avoid chlorine bleach (sodium hypochlorite) and products containing it. Use oxygen bleach instead and unbleached paper products.

- Stay away from pesticides or fungicides that contain chlorine, especially weed killers, such as 2,4-D, which are found in most fertilizers and weed killers, and are commonly used by commercial lawn services. Avoid flea sprays for pets that contain permethrin.

- Make coffee using unbleached (brown) coffee filters or ones that were bleached in nonchlorine bleach.

- In case of occupational exposure to pesticides or other toxins, launder work clothes in a separate load.

We realize that making these changes overnight would be a daunting and overwhelming task. On the other hand, being aware of the problems in our environment and making small changes over time will lead to larger and more profound changes. We know because we've done it in our own lives. And we're still not there yet.

## Last Word

*I started making changes one at a time. Some changes require a single switch in method or action; other changes require an ongoing effort. I started replacing kitchenware years ago, buying glass refrigerator dishes and bakeware to replace plastic and aluminum ones, one piece at a time. Now, I rarely use plastic bags, wrap, or containers. I won't say never, but rarely.*

*I waited three years to be able to spend a hundred dollars on an entire stainless cookware set to replace the Teflon stuff I'd started with. In the meantime, I shopped at thrift stores to replace one pan or pot at a time.*

*But changing how I clean the house and my body was a progression of changes that took very little time and saved me a chunk from my budget. It was just a matter of replacing one product with an alternative and then getting used to the new routine around that alternative product.*

*Change is rarely easy or simple, but good changes can save our lives!*

—D'Ann S., breast cancer survivor

# CHAPTER 5

# NUTRIENT SUFFICIENCIES AND EFFICIENCIES

*The doctor of the future will no longer treat the human frame with drugs, but rather will cure and prevent disease with nutrition.*

—Thomas Edison

> CHAPTER GOAL: Understand what your own nutritional deficiencies are and correct them, using whole foods and high-quality nutritional supplements

Scientists and medical professionals have known for quite some time that breast cancer and other cancers occur as a result of uncontrolled cell proliferation. But exactly what causes this out-of-control growth still remains a bit of a mystery that is being pieced together, study by study. What we do know is that many carcinogens do their dirty work by damaging our DNA. The greater our exposure to carcinogens, the greater the potential for DNA damage that can lead to cancer.

When our DNA becomes damaged, our genes begin to mutate, or change form. For example, when a gene that helps control cell division is damaged, the cell can no longer control the process effectively. When carcinogens silence the genes that are designed to protect us from cancer (for example, the p53, or "tumor suppressor," gene), we will stop benefiting from their protection. When the genes that regulate the normal life cycle of a cell malfunction, the normal process of cell death, or apoptosis, can be impeded.

So it would be fair to say that one of a cell's top priorities is to protect its DNA. Our cells accomplish this aim by maintaining a good stockpile of repair enzymes to reverse damage and by having an ample supply of antioxidants to reduce oxidative stress. To satisfy these needs, cells must have the right nutrients at the right time. The cell membrane has the job of making sure that these nutrients gain entry into the cell as required and that toxins are eliminated as necessary.

In this chapter we'll discuss those nutrients that seem to be most intimately related to protecting cellular DNA and performing other functions essential to preventing cancer. We'll also discuss a few nutrients that, in excess, can raise the risk of recurrence, and we'll share information on the safest and most effective forms of these nutrients.

We like to think of nutrition as you might think of a bank account. A sedentary lifestyle, poor sleep, and poor eating habits are the withdrawals that rob nutritional reserves. Deposits come from eating whole, nutrient-dense foods that replenish reserves. The interest is the strength and vitality that come from smart investing. At the end of the chapter we'll give you some specific ways to discover the status of your own nutritional "bank account."

# Nutrients to the Rescue

Literally thousands of studies have uncovered a clear and distinct relationship between vital nutrients and cancer risk. One influential study (Ramesha et al. 1990) provides a powerful example. A powerful carcinogen known as DMBA was given to a group of female rats. Then the rats were given none, one of four, two of four, three of four, or all of four nutrients: the minerals selenium and magnesium, and vitamins C and A. The results were truly astonishing. When no nutrients were administered, *all* of the rats developed breast cancer. When *one* of the nutrients was given, 46.4 to 57.1 percent of the rats developed tumors, depending on the nutrient. When two of the nutrients were given in combination, the tumor incidence further decreased to 25.9 to 34.6 percent, depending on the combination. Administration of nutrients in groups of threes resulted in still further reduction of tumor incidences, approximately 16 to 23.1 percent. And when all four nutrients were given together, tumor incidence dropped to 12 percent. Remember, our DNA is 99 percent identical to that of rats. Nutrition is power!

## Professor Ames's Triage Theory

A professor of biochemistry at the University of California, Bruce Ames (2006) is one of the most frequently cited scientists in the world, with over five hundred publications and several dozen awards to his name. Ames has been working on a theory connecting micronutrient intake, cancer risk, and other degenerative diseases. Known as Ames's "triage theory," it suggests, among other things, that optimizing intake of the approximately forty essential nutrients (vitamins, minerals, amino acids, and fatty acids) leads to a reduction in chronic, degenerative diseases, including cancer. Let's take a look at some of the nutrients that Ames and others consider to be the most critical ones for keeping cancer at bay. Keep in mind, however, that there's just no substitute for getting *all* of the nutrients you need, *all* of the time, and a nutrient-dense, Eating for Health diet is your foundation for accomplishing this.

# Iodine: Mammary Gland Gatekeeper?

The title of this section is based on a 2005 article, "Is Iodine a Gatekeeper of the Integrity of the Mammary Gland?" (Aceves, Anguiano, and Delgado), in which a strong case is made for the role of iodine in "contributing to the integrity of the normal mammary gland" through its function as both an antioxidant and an antiproliferative agent. In fact, Dr. David Brownstein, author of *Iodine: Why You Need It, Why You Can't Live Without It*, goes so far as to state:

> The chance of a woman having invasive breast cancer sometime during her life is now one in seven. The single most important nutrient to halt this progression is iodine. In fact inadequate breast iodine levels have been associated with the development of breast cancer in both animals and humans, while iodine supplementation has been shown to cause cancer cells to shift into apoptosis or programmed cell death. I have no doubt one of the reasons we are seeing such an epidemic of breast cancer is due to iodine deficiency. (pers. comm.)

There's a wealth of data to back him up. For example, in Japan, where the population consumes approximately 14 milligrams of iodine daily from seaweed, women have one of the lowest breast cancer rates in the world (Kawamura and Sobue 2005).

Investigators observed the same phenomenon experimentally in rats, when the animals were given a potent carcinogen and then some were treated with various forms of iodine and thyroid hormone. The researchers found that the rats that received the treatment experienced almost 41 percent fewer tumors (Aceves, Anguiano, and Delgado 2005). This is a big difference!

Human studies identifying the connection between iodine deficiency and breast tumors actually date back over forty years (Eskin et al. 1967), but have been slow to come to the attention of the public. One did recently, however. Two groups of breast cancer patients were studied who had undergone biopsy but not had surgery yet. One group was given iodine and the other a placebo. Next, breast tissue was analyzed and compared after surgery. Results showed that "although tumor size did not differ between groups, a significantly lower proliferation and increased apoptotic rate [cell death] were observed in tumors from women supplemented with iodine" (Vega-Riveroll et al. 2008).

What happened exactly? In a nutshell:

- Tumor cells replicated more slowly.

- Tumor cells died more quickly.

- The growth factor known as VEGF (vascular endothelial growth factor) was diminished.

- Blood vessels grown expressly to "feed" the tumor in a process known as angiogenesis were fewer in number.

Interestingly, iodine levels began to fall precipitously in the United States in the 1970s, as breast cancer rates began to rise. In fact, iodine levels declined a full 50 percent between 1971 and 2000 (Caldwell et al. 2008). This drop began in earnest when bakers started substituting bromide for potassium iodate (a form of iodine) as a dough conditioner in baking; some manufacturers added bromide to sodas; and others used bromide in medications, flame retardants, pesticides, or some combination of these compounds. Since bromide competes with iodine for absorption (as do the elements fluoride and chorine), it's easy to become deficient in iodine when our bodies are saturated with bromide, fluoride, and chlorine from food, water, and personal care products on a daily basis.

## Assessing Your Iodine Status

The best way to discover whether you are iodine deficient is to take an *iodine loading test* (a large dose of iodine), which a holistic practitioner can provide. This test, developed by Dr. Guy Abraham, measures the amount of iodine you expel in your urine. When the body has a sufficient supply of iodine, the excess is excreted. Higher levels of iodine in urine signify lower or nonexistent degrees of iodine deficiency. In Helayne's practice, she has yet to find a woman who does not test as deficient in iodine.

## Sources of Iodine

Concentrated food sources of iodine are sea vegetables, yogurt, organic milk, eggs, and fish, including shellfish. We enjoy experimenting with various types of seaweed. Sea vegetables are delicious and easy to add to your diet. A few strips of kombu or wakame, boiled in water, make a simple broth to which you can add other ingredients. Adding chipped dulse to a pot of beans or other legumes boosts both nutrition and flavor. Dulse flakes, available in natural groceries, are a tasty addition when sprinkled on salads or sandwiches, while toasted nori sheets make a great snack. Toasted and crumbled nori can also be great sprinkled on popcorn.

## Note of Caution about Iodine

If you have an autoimmune thyroid disease (for example, Hashimoto's thyroiditis), you may be more susceptible to problems that can arise from excessive iodine consumption. It is very important to consult with your holistic health care practitioner before starting on a supplementation program.

# Vitamin D: Not Just for Bones Anymore

If awards were given out for vitamins, vitamin D would certainly win in the popularity category. The darling of the medical and nutritional world for the past several years, this hormonelike vitamin has a host of tasks: it helps regulate calcium utilization, exerts a direct effect on both insulin and blood pressure, and helps protect bone integrity. But we're interested in its role in maintaining healthy immunity and in normalizing cellular differentiation to help lower the risk of an occurrence or recurrence of breast cancer.

## Cell Differentiation

*Differentiation* is the process by which cells develop specialized characteristics. As they mature, cells differentiate to take on specific roles in the body; for example, a breast cell carries out its tasks once it is well differentiated. When cells are well differentiated, they tend not to divide as quickly. To maintain good health, keeping cells dividing at the appropriate rate is a top priority, because an overproliferation of cells with damaged DNA can lead to cancer. Vitamin D inhibits this process of overproliferation and stimulates healthy differentiation of cells (Holick 2004).

## Immunity

Vitamin D is also a powerful immune system modulator; for example, we know that vitamin D is essential for activating specialized immune cells known as *T cells* (Rode von Essen et al. 2010). You'll find more about T cells and other immune cells in chapter 7.

## Protection against Breast Cancer

In population studies, vitamin D also exhibits a strong association with lowering breast cancer risk. For example, researchers who studied women in the first National Health and Nutrition Examination Survey (NHANES I) found that sunlight exposure and vitamin D intake were connected to a lower risk of breast cancer about twenty years later in life (John et al. 1999).

In 2007, Cedric Garland, a prominent vitamin D researcher, published the results of two *case-control studies* (studies that examine patients who already have a disease to see if they have characteristics that differ from those of people without the disease). Garland and his colleagues noted that women with a 25-hydroxyvitamin D blood level of 52 nanograms per milliliter had half the chance of developing breast cancer as women with $D_3$ levels lower than 13 nanograms per milliliter.

Unfortunately, most American women are vitamin D deficient, a fact we have seen repeatedly in our own practices. Women with the lowest levels tend to be older, darker skinned, and heavier (vitamin D is stored in body fat, making it less readily available for active use) (Arunabh et al. 2003). What's more, women who use sunscreen every day or go outside infrequently are also at a high risk of deficiency, as are women on cholesterol-lowering drugs, since cholesterol is required for vitamin D synthesis. The latitude where you live also affects your body's ability to convert sunlight into vitamin D. Many parts of the United States (particularly latitudes north of the 37th parallel north) do not get sufficient ultraviolet B (UVB) rays during the winter months due to the angle of the sun at this time, so supplementing with vitamin $D_3$ (cholecalciferol) during the winter may be particularly critical.

Most, but not all, large-scale studies show that vitamin D plays a role in lowering the risk of breast cancer. But having a reduced risk of a disease does not guarantee that you will never get it. It merely lowers your chances. As summed up in the *American Journal of Public Health*, "The majority of studies found a protective relationship between sufficient vitamin D status and lower risk of cancer. The evidence suggests that efforts to improve vitamin D status ... could reduce cancer incidence and mortality at low cost, with few or no adverse effects" (Garland et al. 2006).

## Assessing Your Vitamin D Status

There are two forms of vitamin D found in blood: 25-hydroxyvitamin D (25[OH]D) is the so-called "storage" form of D, while 1,25-hydroxyvitamin D is considered the "active" form. Most experts agree that a blood test for 25(OH)D is the best way to assess your vitamin D status, but not all agree on what ideal blood levels are. So-called "healthy levels" can range from 40 nanograms per milliliter to 125 nanograms per milliliter, depending on whom you consult. Since each of us is biochemically unique, we need different levels of vitamin D depending on age, health status, vitamin A sufficiency, calcium status, and a host of other factors.

## Our Perspective on Vitamin D

While adequate vitamin D levels are important to good health, it's equally important to guard against vitamin D toxicity and avoid its use in conjunction with specific conditions. People with *sarcoidosis,* an autoimmune condition, should not supplement with vitamin D, for example, because it can exacerbate this condition. Generalized vitamin D toxicity can also cause major health difficulties for people with liver or kidney issues. In addition, excessive D supplementation can boost levels of blood calcium too high, a condition known as *hypercalcemia*. As with all supplements, more is not necessarily better!

We support the judicious use of sunlight whenever possible and modest supplementation of vitamin $D_3$ (cholecalciferol), if needed, combined with regular monitoring of your 25(OH)D level and serum calcium levels. A blood level of 50 to 80 nanograms per milliliter of 25(OH)D is, in our opinion, worth aiming for. Always be sure to work with a knowledgeable health practitioner to optimize and monitor your vitamin D levels.

# Vitamin C

*Ascorbic acid* (vitamin C) is well known as the "anti-scurvy" vitamin. Many of us remember learning in high-school biology that old-time sailors were infamous for getting this dreadful disease, caused by an extreme vitamin C deficiency, until Scottish surgeon James Lind uncovered the cure in citrus fruits.

Many of us also remember Linus Pauling, Nobel laureate and pioneering researcher on the health effects of vitamin C. Some may even be familiar with his famous trials in the 1970s and 1980s with Dr. Ewan Cameron. These trials suggested that large intravenous doses of vitamin C helped increase survival time and improve quality of life for terminal cancer patients (Cameron and Pauling 1976). Since then, the use of intravenous vitamin C as a cancer treatment has been hotly debated. But what has not been controversial is the importance of vitamin C as a helpful cancer preventative and overall contributor to health and longevity.

How does it work? Ed proposes three prevention mechanisms concerning vitamin C:

- Its intake can stimulate the immune system by increasing NK (natural killer) cell activity.

- It is a powerful antioxidant and therefore may inhibit carcinogenesis.

- It has an antihistamine effect. In animal studies, histamine and inflammation have long been associated with tumor promotion (Scolnik, Rubio, and Caro 1985).

Studies on the relationship between vitamin C and breast cancer risk have, thus far, produced a hodgepodge of results. Several studies found no association, while some noteworthy studies found a compelling relationship. In the Nurses' Health Study, for example, premenopausal women who obtained about 200 milligrams per day of vitamin C from foods had less than half the risk of breast cancer of women who consumed only 70 milligrams per day (Zhang et al. 1999). The FDA's current recommended daily allowance (RDA) for women, based on the amount needed to prevent scurvy, is a meager 75 milligrams per day, possibly lulling us into a false sense of security about this critical nutrient.

## Our Perspective on Vitamin C

Vitamin C does its best work when consumed in a whole-food form, complete with the bioflavonoids that are part of the vitamin C family. Flavonoids are a class of plant compounds that not only act as antioxidants on their own but also boost the power of vitamin C and other nutrients. Citrus bioflavonoids actually help increase vitamin C absorption while working synergistically with it.

So, when it comes to vitamin C for breast cancer prevention, we encourage you to eat plenty of vitamin C- and bioflavonoid-rich fruits and vegetables. We recommend organic red peppers, strawberries, oranges, lemons, papayas, broccoli, and kale as a great starting point.

The website of World's Healthiest Foods (whfoods.com) contains a complete listing and serves as a great reference for all health concerns, plus it's one of our favorite sites. As this encyclopedic resource informs us, vitamin C is highly susceptible to degradation from air, water, and variations in temperature. Any type of cooking, freezing, thawing, or canning (even steaming) can cause vitamin C–rich produce to lose some of its potency. Handle with care!

For additional breast cancer protection, we recommend an additional 1 to 3 grams of vitamin C each day in supplement form. Buffered C with at least 500 to 750 milligrams of bioflavonoids is best.

# Selenium

The mineral selenium is known to be another one of the most effective nutrients for natural protection from breast cancer and other cancers as well. Unfortunately, not many of us obtain the recommended dose of 200 micrograms a day.

Selenium is widely known as a scavenger of free radicals (which result from unwelcome chemical reactions in the body) and is even more powerful when combined with vitamin E. Furthermore, selenium seems to prevent damaged DNA from replicating, thus helping to stop cancer before it can start developing, according to Dr. James Howenstine (2008).

Selenium is also necessary for manufacturing *glutathione*, the body's own natural antioxidant. Found in every one of your cells, glutathione helps you remain healthy by keeping free radicals in check, detoxifying metals and carcinogens, helping to transport amino acids into cells, and much more. Malnutrition, stress, and toxicity can all deplete our glutathione levels, putting our immune systems at risk. It's no wonder that selenium is regarded as an anticancer nutrient.

Hundreds of studies confirm this, beginning in the late 1950s and ongoing today. In 2006 an entire issue of *Biomedical and Life Sciences* was devoted to examining selenium as an anticancer agent, its authors (Combs and Lü) concluding:

> Most epidemiological studies have shown inverse associations of selenium (Se) status and cancer risk; almost all experimental animal studies have shown that supranutritional exposures of Se can reduce tumor yield; and each of the limited number of clinical intervention trials conducted to date has found Se treatment to be associated with reductions in cancer risks.

## Food Sources of Selenium

The amount of selenium in soil has steadily declined over the years, reflected in diminishing levels of selenium in fruits and vegetables. Therefore the amount of selenium in food fluctuates depending on where it was grown. And while selenium can induce toxic effects in very large doses, most of us are actually deficient in this mineral. Good sources of selenium include mushrooms, organic egg yolks, seafood, poultry, whole grains, broccoli, asparagus, and Brazil nuts. In fact, eating just a few Brazil nuts a day will meet your daily requirement. So crack open a few Brazil nuts and wash them down with a glass of vitamin C–rich orange or tomato juice!

Should you decide to supplement with selenium, the Life Extension Foundation (www.lef.org), a well-respected source of nutritional information and online supplement retailer, recommends *Se-methylselenocysteine* (SeMSC), a naturally occurring, organic selenium compound found in garlic and broccoli, whose effectiveness has been established both in vitro and in vivo (El-Bayoumy et al. 2006).

# Zinc

Zinc is another essential mineral that contributes to many bodily functions, informing our senses of taste and smell, maintaining skin health, and keeping the male reproductive system running smooothly. Zinc also contributes to a healthy immune system, by supporting the thymus gland and assisting in the production of T lymphocytes (T cells). There seems to be a direct relationship between zinc deficiency (identified through blood and hair samples) and both breast and ovarian cancer (Memon et al. 2007). The breasts have a unique relationship with zinc, since the production of breast milk requires substantial quantities of zinc. One study published in *Genes and Nutrition* noted that "dysregulated mammary gland zinc metabolism has recently been implicated in breast cancer transition, progression, and metastasis" (Kelleher, Seo, and Lopez 2009). (*Metastasis* is tumor spread; a secondary tumor that can result is also called a metastasis.)

Because zinc is so important to maintaining immune-system health, and given the studies indicating its importance to female health, it is reasonable to consider adding foods high in zinc to the diet. The RDA for nonpregnant, nonlactating women is 15 milligrams per day. Zinc is plentiful in a wide variety of foods, for example, calf liver, pumpkin seeds, cremini mushrooms, spinach, Swiss chard, collard greens, and yogurt.

If your zinc levels are especially low, you may wish to consider supplementation. You can measure your zinc levels with a blood test or a simple, oral zinc "challenge test." Discuss this possibility with your nutritionist or holistic practitioner.

# Magnesium

Magnesium, one of our essential macrominerals, is critical for heart and bone health. Approximately 65 percent of the magnesium in our bodies is stored in our bones and teeth, while the other 35 percent is located in bodily fluids, inside cells, and in muscle tissue.

Used by the ancient Romans as a laxative (and still used that way today), magnesium, in recent years, has been shown to be an effective and valuable adjunct to treatment for a variety of health issues, and to help reduce cancer risk as well. As far back as 1970 (Aleksandrowicz et al.), it was known that *hypomagnesia*, too little magnesium in the body, seemed to be an important risk factor for cancer.

Equally important was a then-new study demonstrating that adding magnesium into the diet of rats actually helped a specific type of benign tumor, known as "desmoid," to disappear completely (Hunt and Belanger 1972). In 1986, a landmark study published in *Anticancer Research* (Durlach et al.) boldly proclaimed, "Magnesium deficiency seems to be carcinogenic." While the mechanism is not entirely clear, we do know that magnesium is responsible for participating in over three hundred enzymatic reactions in the body: like selenium it is involved in producing glutathione, our internal antioxidant; it is also essential in the manufacture of *ATP*, the molecule that provides energy for nearly all metabolic processes. In other words, magnesium facilitates a lot of healthy actions and reactions!

## Sources of Magnesium

The current recommended daily value for adult females is 320 milligrams per day, which is not hard to get when nutritionally available sources are so rich in magnesium content. Dark-green, leafy vegetables, such as Swiss chard and spinach (each providing around 150 milligrams per 1 cup serving), are an excellent source of magnesium, as are pumpkin seeds, blackstrap molasses, whole grains, nuts, and bananas. But stress and numerous medications, such as birth control pills, deplete magnesium stores, so supplementation may be advisable. If you choose this route, make sure to use a highly absorbable form of magnesium, such as magnesium glycinate, taurate, or citrate. Magnesium is nontoxic even in large amounts, so it's virtually impossible to take too much. But should you find that the amount you are taking has a laxative effect, cut back until that issue is resolved. About 300 to 400 milligrams a day works well for most people. Some companies now offer magnesium as a transdermal gel or spray oil, bypassing the potential problems inherent with oral supplementation. We have had good luck with these formulations and have seen them work well in our practices. Another option is the traditional Epsom salts (magnesium sulfate) bath, which allows magnesium to be absorbed through the skin while you take a leisurely soak in the tub.

# Other Cancer-Protective Nutrients

The nutrients we've discussed are among the most important for breast cancer defense but certainly do not constitute an exhaustive list. Numerous studies also demonstrate a potent protective role for beta-carotene, vitamin E, vitamin K, and several others. By "eating the rainbow" of vegetables and fruits, plus nuts, seeds, healthy grains, oils, antibiotic-free, hormone-free protein, and the previously mentioned booster foods from the Eating for Health plan, you will get a beneficial dose of all essential nutrients. Enjoy!

## Questionable Dosages

Although most of the approximately forty known nutrients have an extremely wide margin of safety, we're concerned about a few of them when it comes to breast cancer. According to current research, the ones that seem to cause problems or have the potential to do so are iron, copper, and synthetic folic acid.

### IRON

The mineral iron is required for the health and survival of all cells and tissues. The major mineral component of hemoglobin, iron plays a pivotal role in helping to circulate oxygen throughout the body. But, in excess, iron can be as toxic as other heavy metals (such as mercury and lead), because like them, it can produce an excess of free-radical activity that can cause tissue damage (as mentioned earlier, free radicals are atoms or molecules that cause cellular injury).

We tend to get a lot of iron in our commercial food supply, because federal law mandates "fortifying" flour with this mineral. Indeed, at one point several years ago, a magnet could pick up a well-known breakfast cereal due to its high iron content! Iron is also included in many multivitamin products.

People with either diagnosed or undiagnosed cancer tend to have higher levels of iron in their bodies. We suggest getting a blood test that looks at your *ferritin* and *TIBC* (total iron-binding capacity) levels, two measures of iron in the body. Try to keep your levels in the lower half of the normal range without letting yourself become anemic. You can start by making sure that your daily multivitamin does not contain iron, particularly if you're no longer menstruating or are male. Also avoid eating iron-rich foods with citrus or other produce that's high in vitamin C, because vitamin C enhances absorption of iron. In our practices we suggest taking extra vitamin E (600 to 1200 milligram mixed tocopherols), which protects against excess iron in the system. In *Natural Strategies for Cancer Patients*, Dr. Russell Blaylock (2003) also recommends black tea; the flavonoids quercetin, rutin, hesperidin, and naringenin (think apples, onions, citrus fruits, apricots, cherries, and buckwheat); and the supplement inositol phosphate-6 (IP-6) as effective iron *chelators* (chemicals that facilitate the removal of metals from the body).

## COPPER

Copper, like iron, can exhibit two different faces. On the one hand, it's a vital component of dozens of enzymes in the body. It helps out with cellular energy production and supports connective tissue health, and is a critical ingredient of one of the body's powerful endogenous (made internally) antioxidants known as superoxide dismutase. Copper also helps in the formation of new blood vessels, and there's the rub: tumors need blood vessels in order to grow. In the angiogenesis process (in Latin *angio* means "blood vessel," and *genesis* means "to create"), a tumor sends out specialized chemical signals to help it build a complex of blood vessels for transporting nutrients and enzymes to facilitate its growth and development.

Dr. Judah Folkman, surgeon and scientist, first documented this phenomenon in the 1960s (Cooke 2001). His discoveries eventually led to the development of the cancer drug Avastin (bevacizumab), designed to cut off this overzealous network of blood vessels. Meanwhile, other researchers determined that the specialized enzymes that promote angiogenesis depend on the mineral copper to function appropriately (Brem et al. 1990). And it turns out that breast cancer patients often exhibit elevated levels of copper, a sign that the tumor is attempting to sustain the process of angiogenesis (Zowczak et al. 2001).

To translate this information into a risk reduction strategy, we recommend keeping your copper levels at the low end of normal to help prevent recurrence of a tumor. When copper levels are reduced, an incipient tumor has greater difficulty forming new blood vessels to take in nutrients and oxygen. According to Dr. Sofia Merajver, quoted in the *Journal of the National Cancer Institute* (Vanchieri 2000), "There is a window at which copper levels are low enough to block angiogenesis, but not so low that they harm more essential cellular processes."

Blood tests, such as for serum copper and *ceruloplasmin* (a protein produced by the liver that binds copper for transport in the blood), can help you ascertain how much copper you are carrying around. If it is too high, you'll want to avoid high-copper foods, such as shellfish, chocolate, calf liver, sesame seeds, and cashews. Make sure your multivitamin is copper free, avoid copper cookware, and filter your water to avoid taking in copper from household pipes. If none of these strategies brings your copper levels down sufficiently, you can employ both nutritional and pharmaceutical chelating strategies to reduce copper levels. You'll need to consult a nutritional or medical specialist to implement these strategies.

## FOLIC ACID

*Folic acid*, also known as *folate* or *folacin*, is one of the B-complex vitamins widely known for its key role in preventing neural tube defects during pregnancy. The terms "folic acid" and "folate" are sometimes used interchangeably, although *folate* is the natural compound found in food such as green, leafy vegetables, while *folic acid* is a synthetic form of the vitamin found in supplements.

Aside from its role in pregnancy, folate also plays an essential role in helping all cells divide and reproduce exactly as they're meant to. Because of folate's key contributions to the normal process of cell division, folate deficiency has been associated with not only breast cancer but also cancers of the cervix, colon and rectum, lung, esophagus, brain, and pancreas (Maruti, Ulrich, and White 2009).

But folic acid, the synthetic form of folate, can be a double-edged sword. When people ingest large doses of folic acid in fortified cereals, breads, and pastas, for example, they are getting more folic acid than the body can handle, and it is *not* chemically identical to the natural folates found in green, leafy vegetables and other foods. In fact Dr. Barry Boyd (2010) believes that synthetic folic acid can interfere with the proper metabolism of natural folate. Other experts are convinced that excess synthetic folic acid can act like a "fertilizer" in a garden of cells, supporting the growth of cancer cells as well as normal cells (Cristiana Paul, MS, Nutrition Science, pers. comm.).

To be safe, make sure your multivitamin uses folate or folinic acid, a natural form of folate. And remember to stay away from fortified, processed grains, because they will not support your health under any circumstances.

# Prescription Drugs and Nutrient Depletion

A critical matter that's often overlooked by medical professionals and consumers alike is the profound effect that pharmaceutical drugs can have on the absorption, utilization, and excretion of nutrients. Drug-induced nutrient depletion can lead to further health challenges, because your cells need all of the vital nutrients all of the time. Be sure to discuss with your nutritionist or integrative physician how you can compensate for any deficiencies your medications may be causing.

# COMMON DRUG-INDUCED NUTRIENT DEPLETIONS

| Prescription Drug Category | Nutrients Depleted |
|---|---|
| *Antibiotics* | |
| antibiotics (general) amoxicillin, penicillin, cephalexin | Friendly intestinal flora, B vitamins, Vitamin K, Vitamin C |
| tetracycline antibiotics | Friendly intestinal flora, Calcium, Magnesium, Iron, Zinc, $B_6$, $B_{12}$ |
| *Anticonvulsants* | |
| phenobarbital and barbiturates | Vitamin D, Vitamin K, Calcium, Folate, Biotin |
| Dilantin (phenytoin) | Vitamin $B_1$, Vitamin $B_{12}$, Biotin, Folate, Vitamin D, Calcium, Vitamin K |
| *Antidepressants* | |
| tricyclic antidepressants: Elavil (amitriptyline), doxepin, clomimpramine, Tofranil (imipramine) | Coenzyme Q10, Vitamin $B_2$ |
| selective serotonin reuptake inhibitors (SSRIs): Prozac (fluoxetine), Zoloft (sertraline) | Melatonin |
| *Antidiabetic drugs* | |
| sulfonylureas: Micronase, Diabeta (both glyburide), biguanides | Coenzyme Q10, Vitamin E |
| Glucophage (metformin) | Coenzyme Q10, Vitamin E, Folate |
| *Anti-inflammatory drugs* | |
| Tegretol (carbamazepine) | Vitamin E, Folate, Biotin |
| Mysoline (primidone) | Folate, Biotin, Vitamin D, Vitamin K |
| valproic acid | Folate, Carnitine |
| *Birth Control Pills* | |
| all types | Magnesium, Vitamin $B_2$, Vitamin C, Zinc, Folate, and possibly Vitamin $B_1$, $B_3$, $B_6$, $B_{12}$ |
| *Statins* | |
| all types | Coenzyme Q10 |

Adapted, with permission, from Designs for Health Ltd.

*Note: This is just a partial list. For a complete reference on drug-induced nutrient depletions, see* The Nutritional Cost of Prescription Drugs *by Ross Pelton and James LaValle, or* The A–Z Guide to Drug-Herb-Vitamin Interactions *by Alan Gaby et. al.*

# (Almost) Everything You Wanted to Know about Supplements (but Were Afraid to Ask)

We realize that the subject of supplements is very confusing for many people. The following are some common questions our clients have asked about supplements over the years.

## What's in a Label?

Today, most multinutrients offer either an RDA or a percentage of daily value on the label as a general nutrition guideline for consumers. The underlying concept is that these allowances should prevent deficiency diseases associated with each nutrient. For example, as discussed previously, 75 milligrams of vitamin C is the amount deemed necessary to prevent scurvy but not the amount that nutritionists think is necessary for optimal health. What's more, such generalizations do not work for some segments of the population, because of biochemical individuality, a concept introduced by biochemist Roger Williams, who first described how differences in individual anatomy, physiology, and genetics determine individual nutritional requirements.

> **TIP:** A poorly formulated supplement shows "100% DV" of each nutrient on the label. We recommend against this type of supplement, because quality manufacturers know that some nutrients are used up more quickly than others (for example, the B vitamins) and some daily values (DVs) are set at unrealistically low levels (for example, vitamin C). On the other hand, some nutrients may be toxic at doses above the RDA (for example, vitamin A and iron). A high-quality multinutrient will take all of this into account in providing a formula that reflects a practical understanding of how nutrients act in the body.

# How Do I Know What Form of the Nutrient Is Best?

All nutrients come in many forms. Please keep two basic principles in mind: First, you'll want a nutrient that's in a form that's as close to the way nature made it as possible. The simple truth is that synthetic products are far less expensive and have a longer shelf life than natural substances. As such, they are the darlings of low-price chain stores and many pharmacies. Look for a brand that says "food based" or "100% whole food." That way, you are getting not only the nutrient but also the cofactors, enzymes, bioflavonoids, and other phytochemicals that help the nutrient perform its job better.

Second, we suggest familiarizing yourself with nutrients that belong to "families" and understanding that ingesting only one "member" of the family can cause problems. An excellent example is vitamin E, which actually consists of a large cast of characters: first, the tocopherols—alpha, beta, delta, and gamma—and then the tocotrienols—also alpha, beta, delta and gamma. Ideally, your multinutrient label will say "mixed tocopherols" or "mixed tocopherols and tocotrienols." An isolated form of one part of a nutrient can easily throw the other parts off balance.

It's also useful to know whether the nutrient is in its active or precursor form. In other words, can your body use it just the way it is, or does the nutrient need to go through some sort of conversion process? Vitamin $B_6$, for example, is known as pyridoxal-5-phosphate in its active, ready-to-be-metabolized form. Only higher-quality brands will invest the resources to provide the active forms of nutrients when possible.

Finally, if you seek out supplements as part of your breast-cancer protection plan, be sure that the form you choose matches the form used in the research studies showing benefit. For example, selenium comes in many forms, but Se-methylselenocysteine (SeMSC) is the form that has shown the most promise in recent studies for cancer prevention (Smith et al. 2004). Avoid multinutrients that do not divulge the form of the nutrient you are being asked to take!

# *How Do I Identify a High-Quality Supplement?*

If you plan to take supplements, it is important to make sure that you are getting what your body needs. Unfortunately this is not always the case. Here are a few of the most critical of several issues to consider when purchasing supplements.

## BIOAVAILABILITY

A nutrient is only as good as your ability to absorb it. So it's good to get a handle on what makes some forms more absorbable than others. Remember, the closer to real food your formula is, the more familiar it will feel to your body. That said, there are a few other basic principles. Minerals, for example, are notoriously hard for the body to absorb in both food and supplement form. Albion Labs, a leader in the nutritional supplement field, estimates that typical absorption rates for minerals range from 10 to 45 percent (quoted in Bauman 2009). The following chart illustrates some common nutrient forms and can serve as a guide to preferable ones.

| Nutrient | Look for |
|---|---|
| Vitamin A | Mixed carotenoids |
| Vitamin $B_1$ | Thiamine HCl |
| Vitamin $B_{12}$ | Methylcobalamin |
| Vitamin D | Cholecalciferol |
| Folate | Folate, Metafolin, MTHF |
| Vitamin E | Mixed tocopherols, mixed tocotrienols |
| Vitamin K | $K_1$ and $K_2$ |
| Calcium | Citrate, ascorbate |
| Magnesium | Glycinate, taurate, citrate, aspartate |
| Selenium | Se-methylselenocysteine, selenomethionine |
| Zinc | Citrate, gluconate |

# NUMBER OF NUTRIENTS INCLUDED

All multinutrient formulas include the basics, but only a high-quality supplement includes trace minerals, which play a vital metabolic function. For example, look for a formula that includes chromium to assist with blood sugar regulation, silicon for hair and nail strength, boron for bone health, and vanadium for insulin sensitivity. These trace minerals are of particular importance since they are scarce in most conventional soils. A good-quality formula includes these trace minerals and more.

# USP CERTIFICATION

A supplement with the USP (U.S. Pharmacopoeia) designation is of the highest quality, indicating that the product has met the following stan-dards: disintegration (you don't want your vitamin pills just sitting in your stomach!), strength, purity, and expiration (when the supplement will no longer meet these standards). Look for the USP symbol to ensure that your supplements have been verified in this fashion.

If you like, you can also request a certificate of analysis from the supplement manufacturer to help ensure quality control and that the label reflects the actual contents. An authentic certificate gives details of the lab where tests were conducted, what was tested, and the lot number of the product tested. This is a good way to be sure the product is free of heavy metals, pesticides, solvents, and other pollutants.

# NO "JUNK" INGREDIENTS

Beware of products with ingredient names you can't pronounce or identify, such as titanium dioxide, stannous chloride, and sodium meta-vanadate, common ingredients in drugstore supplements. Other substances to avoid include all artificial colors and flavors, sugars, artificial sweeteners, and toxic fillers. You might also consider avoiding common allergens, such as lactose, gluten, and cornstarch.

# Questions to Ask Professionals

Some issues around supplements need to be discussed with a professional nutritionist or other holistic practitioner. For example, how do you know what dosage of a nutrient is best for you? Your needs depend on your existing nutritional status, your biochemical makeup, and your individual risk factors for breast cancer. Your practitioner may suggest conducting specific tests that would indicate your need for specific nutrients. This upfront spending can bring large dividends in the long run, because you can then be more judicious in using only those supplements that will provide the most benefit. Other questions to ask your practitioner are:

- *How and when should I take the supplement?*

- *How long should I take the supplement?*

- *What interactions among nutrients do I need to watch for?*

- *What interactions might the supplements have with the herbs or medications I take?*

You will usually get what you pay for. We feel that it is far better to take fewer supplements of better quality than to swallow a trunkful of "junk" supplements that could wind up doing more harm than good.

Keep in mind that supplements, no matter how useful, do not and never will have the same power as nutrient-dense, whole Eating for Health foods. Supplements are meant to be used as an adjunct to a healthy diet, *never* a replacement. Be sure to work with your nutritionist or other holistic practitioner to determine which supplements and dosages are right for your particular situation.

## TO DO

- Be sure to get plenty of all required nutrients, paying special attention to those with documented anticancer activity and making sure to check for nutrient depletions from medications you may be taking.

- Test your iodine and vitamin D levels, because iodine and vitamin D are your superstar protective nutrients. If you are deficient, take steps to raise your levels according to your practitioner's recommendations.

- Avoid nutrients that can cause problems for people who are concerned about cancer recurrence: iron, copper, and synthetic folic acid.

- Quality is more important than quantity when it comes to supplements. Make sure to take both adequate dosages and an absorbable and complete form of your nutrients.

## Last Word

*I was going crazy and spending all my money on every supplement that someone mentioned might be useful. A turning point for me was when I finally decided to invest in knowing what was happening in my body, not my neighbor's or running partner's. Once I started recognizing myself for the unique biochemical being that I am, I could pick and choose the nutrients that made the most sense for me and spend my money on high-quality supplements that I knew were going to help.*

—Carole B., breast cancer survivor

# CHAPTER 6

# GLUCOSE, WEIGHT, AND INSULIN CONTROL

*Sugar is the most hazardous foodstuff in the American diet.*

—Linus Pauling, Nobel laureate

CHAPTER GOAL: Lower glucose and insulin levels

How do you just say no to sugar? With its jolt of sweetness and energy, sugar can be an addictive substance for many of us. What's more, it shows up in different forms in nearly all processed foods, disguised under a variety of names, such as maltodextrin, corn syrup, rice syrup, and dehydrated cane juice, among others. Though these names may not include the word "sugar," make no mistake: they are all forms of sugar. The key is finding strategies to manage your sweet tooth, because sugar has potential effects that just aren't that sweet, as we'll explore in this chapter.

When it comes to cancer, sugar is like gasoline to your car: it's fuel. The notion that sugar "feeds" cancer has been around for almost a century, since Dr. Otto Warburg first determined in 1924 that cancer cells have a way of metabolizing energy that is essentially different from that of noncancerous cells. More-current research has shown that cancer cells are completely reliant on simple sugar to sustain themselves, consuming sugar at a rate "ten to fifty times higher than normal tissues" (Block 2009). What does this mean to you? Feeding your body simple sugars and refined carbohydrates leads to an elevation in blood sugar, also known as "blood glucose," which, effectively, feeds tumors exactly what they need to grow.

But it's not just sugar itself that can harm your body's ecosystem. Ingestion of sugars and simple carbohydrates activates the release of the hormone insulin and its close relative, insulin-like growth factor (IGF-1), both of which are potent cellular-growth promoters in their own right. High levels of blood sugar and insulin have long been known to set the stage for obesity, insulin resistance (prediabetes), and diabetes. It's now becoming crystal clear that they may be doing the same for breast cancer and other cancers as well.

# Dietary Sugar and Cancer: A Sweet Relationship?

Over the past several decades, a vast number of studies have made the connection between sugar and cancer. In fact, a casual search on PubMed (www.ncbi.nlm.nih.gov/pubmed), the online search engine of the U.S. National Library of Medicine, brings up over twenty thousand articles on "glucose and cancer." (For our purposes, "glucose" is another word for sugar.) Clearly, this is an area of intensive investigation!

As you remember from chapter 2, refined carbohydrates, such as white bread, rice, pasta, and many cereals, convert to sugar before they're even swallowed. So keep in mind that when we say "simple" or "refined" carbohydrates, we're also talking, in essence, about sugar. One long-range Swedish study conducted in the late 1980s suggested a link between simple carbs and a common type of breast cancer, *estrogen-receptor positive*, *progesterone-receptor negative* (ER+/PR–). The study analyzed the eating habits of 61,433 women and concluded that "a high carbohydrate intake may increase the risk of developing ER+/PR– breast cancer" (Larsson, Bergkvist, and Wolk 2009).

Put simply, "When we lower blood glucose, we can slow cancer growth," explains nutritionist, cancer specialist, and author Patrick Quillin (2005, 119). A 1985 study (Santisteban et al.) on rats demonstrated this link dramatically. First, aggressive cancer cells were injected into the rats. Then, the rats were fed diets containing assorted quantities of sugar to see which tumors would grow the most rapidly. As anticipated, the rats with the highest levels of blood glucose fared poorly and had the shortest survival time, while those with the lowest glucose levels lived the longest. It makes sense, then, to eat foods that do not disrupt the balance of sugars in your body. To help do this, we check a food's *glycemic index*: a numerical ranking, from 0 to 100, of a food's potential to alter blood glucose levels. Glucose itself is ranked 100 on the index. White bread has a *high* glycemic index, which means it converts to glucose quickly, causing a rapid surge in blood sugar. More-complex carbohydrates, such as whole grains and beans, create a more gradual change in blood glucose and are considered to have a lower glycemic index. Proteins and fats fall low on the glycemic index as well.

As a general rule, leafy vegetables—such as broccoli, lettuce, and cabbage—have a lower glycemic index than root vegetables, like potatoes, carrots, yams, and beets. Most bread, pasta, muffins, cereal, bagels, and *all* other refined grains are carbohydrates with a high glycemic index. Therefore when planning a healthy meal, try to include larger portions of carbohydrates with a low glycemic index and smaller portions of carbohydrates with a high glycemic index.

You may also be familiar with the term *glycemic load*. Glycemic load takes into account the amount of carbohydrates in a *typical portion* of food, so many nutritionists consider it a more accurate measure of a food's effect on blood sugar. For example, a small portion of white rice would have a much lower glycemic load than a plateful of rice. In the Swedish study mentioned previously (Larsson, Bergkvist, and Wolk 2009), women whose dietary intake fell into the highest category of glycemic *load* had an 81 percent increased risk of ER+/PR− tumors.

## Are All Sugars Equal?

Consider the case of high-fructose corn syrup. It actually ranks low on the glycemic index, but don't be fooled. It affects the body in multiple other ways that help create a hospitable environment for cancer. For starters, it is not found in nature; it is manufactured. The process by which it is created uses a "mercury-grade caustic soda" (Dufault et al. 2009) followed by a process known as acid hydrolysis, used to transform cornstarch into corn syrup. Because mercury is actually used to produce this special soda, the soda itself may become tainted and pass along its mercury-contaminated contents to sodas, soups, cereals, salad dressings, and other processed foods. Concerning cancer specifically, we believe that high-fructose corn syrup may:

- Interact with oral contraceptives to elevate insulin levels

- Deplete micronutrient stores

- Elevate blood clotting factors

- Inhibit white blood cell activity

High-fructose corn syrup has also been associated with liver damage (Ouyang et al. 2008).

In a nutshell, although all forms of sugar seem to promote cancer and adversely affect general health, we view this information from different perspectives and to different degrees depending on the type of sugar. High-fructose corn syrup seems to be one of the *most* harmful forms of sugar. Our advice to you is to avoid it at all costs.

## A Hint of Sweetness

Just because we recommend avoiding sugar doesn't mean you need to give up sweetness altogether! Most of us love the taste of sweetness on our palates from time to time. For those occasions, try one of the following sweeteners as a tasty alternative: raw honey, maple syrup (grade B or C is less processed and contains more nutrients than grade A), blackstrap or sorghum molasses, date or palm sugar (low on the glycemic index), stevia, or xylitol. These whole-food sweeteners have a far less dramatic impact on blood glucose because they contain nutrients, one of which is chromium, known for its stabilizing effect on blood sugar. Avoid artificial sweeteners, such as aspartame and Splenda; they are not foods but chemicals, with no known benefit and several suspected harmful effects.

## Weight and Breast Cancer: A Well-Established Association

It has long been known that obesity is influential in the development of breast cancer and negatively affects a patient's prognosis. A variety of large-scale studies have confirmed this association, including the European Prospective Investigation into Cancer and Nutrition (EPIC), which reported a 31 percent greater risk of developing breast cancer in obese women compared to nonobese women (Lahmann, Lissner, and Berglund 2004). What's more, overweight women, particularly those with ER+ tumors, have a higher risk of local lymph node involvement (Verreault et al. 1989). Sadly, it is estimated that up to 50 percent of breast cancer deaths in postmenopausal women in the United States can be attributed to obesity (Petrelli et al. 2002).

Why do we see such an elevation of risk in overweight women? It appears to come down to a constellation of risk factors that converge into what one cancer researcher has dubbed an "oncometabolic state" (Wallace 2010). Features of this oncometabolic state include an abundance of belly fat, elevated glucose or elevated fasting insulin levels (or both), excessive blood lipids (fats), abnormal blood coagulation, and elevated inflammation levels. If these markers sound familiar, it's because they are very similar and, in fact, overlap with markers for a more well-known condition known as *metabolic syndrome*, also known as insulin resistance or prediabetes.

## Elevated Blood Glucose, Elevated Fasting Insulin, or Both

The amount of sugar and simple carbs you ingest will be fairly obvious to you in light of the food choices you make. The level of sugar that circulates in your bloodstream, however, is not nearly as transparent. That's what makes the cycle insidious. Eating sugar causes blood sugar to surge and, subsequently, the hormone insulin to spike. Leaner bodies are better able to move this excess insulin into the cells, where it's intended to be received. In overweight bodies, the tendency is for the excess glucose and insulin to hang around in the bloodstream, causing problems as the cells become increasingly resistant to the action of insulin.

Like gasoline, sugar is highly combustible, which is why it generates intense but short-lived energy. Over time, however, the body's ability to deal with excess sugar diminishes. Eventually this cycle leads to *dysglycemia*, or an imbalance of blood sugar levels and insulin in the body. With dysglycemia, high glucose in the blood leads to high insulin production, which, in turn, can lead to insulin resistance. This is most significant for our purposes because recent data suggest that "hyperinsulinemia [excess insulin] is an independent risk factor for breast cancer and may have a substantial role in explaining the obesity–breast cancer relationship" (Gunter et al. 2009). The literature on this topic clearly serves as a wake-up call to be mindful of blood glucose and insulin control. Fortunately, you have the power to affect these factors because they are exceedingly responsive to dietary changes.

# Assessing Your Glucose and Insulin Status

To assess how your body is handling glucose and insulin, your practitioner can order blood work that examines your fasting glucose and insulin levels, and a protein called *hemoglobin A1c* (HA1c). The fasting glucose number will tell you what your blood glucose level is at a given moment. A range between 70 and 90 is generally considered optimal.

An HA1c level is taken about once every three months, and reflects an average blood-sugar level over that period of time. Be aware that it's possible to have seemingly normal blood glucose levels and still have high levels of insulin in your body. This is important to know so that, if necessary, you can adjust your diet to bring your fasting insulin level into a safe range. This, too, can be assessed through standard laboratory blood work.

Nurse practitioner and diabetes educator Rebecca Murray is assistant clinical professor of nursing at Yale University and runs a medical practice in Groton, Connecticut, where she specializes in diabetes and insulin resistance syndrome. Based on her thousands of patient case studies, Murray suggests (pers. comm.) that an optimal range for HA1c is between 4 and 5.6, and for fasting insulin up to 12 microunits per milliliter. These numbers are based on a twelve-hour fast (ibid.). Keep in mind that if you have a very heavy meal the night before your blood is drawn, your insulin levels could be higher than normal the next morning. So, be sure to test more than once (later that week, for example) to be sure you've got an accurate result.

# Exercise Guidelines

You don't have to train for a triathlon to help reduce your breast cancer risk. Regular exercise of any type cuts your risk of developing the disease and prevents a recurrence. The American Cancer Society (2011a) recommends thirty to sixty minutes of exercise at least five days a week.

All forms of regular exercise can help you reduce your weight. This, in turn, reduces glucose and insulin levels. Exercise is also effective for reducing estrogen levels (which can fuel ER+ tumors, the most common type), and overweight women carry a higher estrogen load than women of a healthy weight (McTiernan et al. 2004).

In fact in 2007, the *Journal of Clinical Oncology* (Pierce et al.) provided an exciting report indicating that increased physical activity, combined with a healthy diet, was associated with an approximately 50 percent reduction in mortality in breast cancer patients.

Whether as a strategy for breast-cancer prevention or for recovery, exercise extends life. Find an exercise program you can commit to; check out your local gym or recreation center and try something new, maybe that spinning class you've been thinking about. Whatever you choose, maintaining an exercise routine will surely reduce your risk of recurrence.

# Diet: How Eating for Health Manages Dysglycemia

In the Eating for Health approach to managing dysglycemia, we recommend a diet that contains approximately:

- 25 to 30 percent of calories from proteins
- 20 to 30 percent of calories from good-quality fats
- 40 to 50 percent of calories from complex carbohydrates

In short, the key to glycemic control is to minimize the amount of refined carbohydrates consumed. As often as this is said, it is hard to hear and truly understand, because breads, pasta, bagels, and pastries are so much a part of our culture.

## Reimagining Breakfast: The Power of Protein

Breakfast is the most important meal of the day; after all, you have fasted all night long. And the most important macronutrient to include in your breakfast is protein. That's because:

- Protein is satiating and, in most people, stabilizes blood sugar for three to four hours.

- Protein stimulates the production of *glucagon*, the hormone that promotes the mobilization and utilization of fat for energy, *not* storage.

87

A high-glycemic bagel, a muffin and coffee, or a bowl of sugary cereal won't provide the protein you need to steady your blood-sugar level; you will find yourself craving carbs again soon after eating such a breakfast, setting up a vicious cycle. If you ignore your hunger and don't eat, your blood sugar can drop too low, setting you up for a wild ride of blood sugar crashes and spikes. You might have a sense of these crashes from symptoms such as headaches, brain fog, irritability, or cravings.

To maintain a balanced blood-sugar level—thereby giving yourself stable energy throughout your day—try to make the time to prepare a balanced meal in the morning. A balanced breakfast includes protein but also provides fat and complex carbohydrates. This means eggs and greens; cottage cheese and fruit; or a protein-based smoothie (we suggest rice or whey protein powder) made with yogurt and fruit, for example.

## Keep Your Life Simple and Your Carbohydrates Complex

This is, indeed, a good rule to live by. But the reverse seems to be the case for many women, whose lives are overcomplex and whose foods are overrefined. Refined or simple carbohydrates include bakery products, pastas, and sugar-containing foods. Unrefined or complex carbohydrates are found in fresh vegetables, fruits, whole cereal grains, legumes, and nuts. Unrefined carbohydrates provide generous amounts of fiber, both soluble (in water) and insoluble. Fiber slows the rate at which glucose from foods is released into the blood and speeds the elimination of the indigestible food and bacterial waste.

## Where Fat Fits

Fats, like protein and carbs, belong in every meal. Choose fats that are mostly monounsaturated, such as those in olives and avocados; healthy saturated fats like coconut oil; or the omega-3 unsaturated fatty acids found in cold-water fish, flaxseeds, and walnuts. Remember that it is not the quantity but the quality of fat that determines its value in the diet. An excess of cooked or processed fats and oils—such as factory-raised animal fats, dairy, and margarine—interferes with the burning of glucose and increases insulin resistance. The essential fatty acids found in fish, seeds, and nuts, on the other hand, and the monounsaturated fatty acids (MUFAs) found in olives, avocados, and their oils tend to slow glucose absorption and balance insulin production, improving insulin sensitivity. Eating a sufficient amount of high-quality dietary fats will also help you feel more satisfied after a meal, which reduces the temptation to snack on refined carbs.

## Micronutrients and Phytonutrients

The previous advice focuses on the macronutrient balances that are most likely to stabilize blood sugar. But for macronutrients to be effective, adequate micronutrients and phytonutrients are needed to produce the necessary enzymes and hormones for everything to work together.

One way to start is by choosing local, organic food. Organic food has been shown to be significantly higher in trace mineral nutrition by a factor of two to ten times when compared to the conventionally grown products generally available in supermarkets (Grinder-Pedersen et al. 2003). If you eat a high proportion of conventional foods from the supermarket and experience the signs and symptoms of dysglycemia, it's likely that you are missing essential vitamins and minerals to support the proper synthesis of insulin and glucagon—most notably chromium, magnesium, and zinc. Likewise, a conventional standard American diet lacks the substances that make cell membranes more sensitive, rather than more resistant, to insulin. To counter this problem, we recommend consuming plenty of essential fatty acids of the omega-3 variety found in flaxseeds, fish, and algae, as well as vitamin E, coenzyme Q10, and lipoic acid.

We have seen people who eat very well and regularly take culinary and medicinal herbs manage this dysglycemic process without multivitamins and minerals because their food is rich in these factors. But we have not seen people who take a variety of well-chosen vitamins, minerals, and herbs succeed in stabilizing blood-sugar levels if their diets include regular infusions of fast foods, sugar, and stimulants like coffee.

## Feed Your Cells Nutritional Superstars

A growing body of scientific research has revealed that many single nutrients, herbs, and foods—the nutritional "superstars"—along with an

Eating for Health diet, provide substantial health benefits to slow and reverse dysglycemia and other inflammatory disorders. While it's possible to supplement any diet with fatty acids, dietary fibers, and vitamins and minerals, we prefer to obtain as many of these nutrients as possible from foods first, supplements second. Here are some suggestions.

## CHILE PEPPERS

Research conducted in Australia has shown that using chile peppers as a flavorful addition to foods allows the body to produce less insulin to transport glucose into cells, preventing an insulin overload (Ahuja et al. 2006). Chile peppers not only lower the amount of insulin required to decrease after-meal blood-sugar levels, but also result in a lower *C-peptide/ insulin quotient*, indicating that the liver's ability to clear insulin has improved. (C-peptide is an indication of how much insulin is being released.) Chile peppers can be used as a versatile flavor enhancer for nearly any kind of recipe, from blended smoothies and cooked dishes to appetizers, sandwiches, and snacks.

## CINNAMON

The world's most ubiquitous spice, cinnamon has historically been used as a glucose-lowering vehicle as well as a flavor enhancer, although its mechanism of action was unclear until recently. In 2000 scientists discovered that the most active compound in cinnamon is a flavonoid called *methylhydroxychalcone polymer* (MHCP), which has been found to improve glucose metabolism twentyfold in fat cells (Jarvill-Taylor, Anderson, and Graves 2001). This is a truly remarkable spice and one that can also serve an anti-inflammatory function, as you'll see in the next chapter.

## OLIVE OIL AND AVOCADOS

Eating avocados and replacing other dietary fats with olive oil may be two of the best, tastiest, and least-known ways to manage blood sugar and insulin (Garg 1998). In addition to being one of the best food sources of monounsaturated fatty acids, avocados also provide B vitamins, magnesium, copper, and manganese in meaningful quantities. Try putting half an avocado in your salad or smoothie daily to get its full beneficial effect.

## LEGUMES AND WHOLE GRAINS

Legumes and whole grains are complex carbohydrates that are loaded with nutrients and high in soluble fiber, which helps keep blood-sugar levels under control (Fung et al. 2002). Whole grains appear to be particularly useful, perhaps because of the generous levels of magnesium they pack. Fiber and magnesium are both associated with a lowered risk of type 2 diabetes (ibid.).

Buckwheat, the grain often used in pancakes and soba noodles, also came to the forefront of blood-sugar control when a Canadian study found that extracts of buckwheat, when fed to diabetic rats, lowered their glucose levels by 12 to 19 percent (Kawa, Taylor, and Przybylski 2003). Buckwheat contains significant amounts of fiber, B vitamins, copper, magnesium, and manganese, as well as moderate amounts of zinc; brown rice does, as well. Beans and legumes are also good sources of the B vitamins, including $B_6$.

## BITTER MELON

A tropical fruit indigenous to Asia, East Africa, and South America, bitter melon (also known as *karela*) can be purchased fresh in Asian markets or in extract form from health food stores. Several studies have shown that it can significantly lower blood glucose levels. Its effect on blood sugar is believed to be due to an increase in the activity of *hexokinase* and *glucokinase*, specialized enzymes that convert sugar into *glycogen*, a storage form of glucose that can be salted away in the liver for later use (Chen, Chan, and Li 2003). Bitter melon is also available in supplement form.

## GYMNEMA SYLVESTRE (GUMAR)

*Gymnema sylvestre* (also called *gumar*) is a tropical plant from the milkweed family with an ancient Sanskrit name that means, literally, "destroyer of sugar." Preliminary clinical research indicates that certain gymnema extracts can reduce blood glucose and HA1c in types 1 and 2 diabetics (Kumar, Mani, and Mani 2010).

## STEVIA (SWEET HERB)

*Stevia* is a noncaloric herb, native to Paraguay, that has been used to sweeten and enhance flavor for hundreds of years. In a small study that compared numerous effects of sucrose, aspartame, and stevia, only stevia reduced insulin levels after meals (Anton et al. 2010).

## CHROMIUM

This essential trace mineral, discovered in 1797 by French chemist Nicolas-Louis Vauquelin, was later found to play a key role in carbohydrate metabolism by helping to create a critical compound called *glucose tolerance factor* (GTF). As the active component of GTF, chromium plays a fundamental role in controlling blood sugar levels. Romaine lettuce, broccoli, onions, and tomatoes are high in chromium, as are nutritional yeast, oysters, liver, whole grains, and potatoes.

Because many people don't eat whole foods, they don't get enough chromium in their diets, due to food-processing methods that remove the naturally occurring chromium from common foods. An adequate intake of chromium for adult women is 20 to 25 micrograms a day, although people with any sort of blood sugar issues may well want to experiment with levels from 100 to 200 micrograms a day, which is still considered extremely safe. A high-quality multinutrient should contain approximately this amount.

# The Rainbow Provides the "Pot of Gold"

Eating for Health is eating from the rainbow. Consuming a wide variety of colorful vegetables, fruits, and other foods on a regular basis provides the widest spectrum of health-giving nutrients and may help us all find our way to the "pot of gold"—our good health. In the process, we will leave behind our blood sugar irregularities and greatly reduce our risk of insulin resistance, diabetes, and breast cancer.

Our list of supernutrients in this chapter is by no means exhaustive. In fact, a varied whole-foods diet, with or without these foods, will provide enormous benefits toward preventing or reversing dysglycemia and maintaining overall health. In addition, please keep in mind that whole fruits (not juice) and, especially, vegetables contain some of the highest levels of vitamins and minerals, as well as large amounts of fiber, of any foods. They also provide a wide range of phytonutrients, which helps us with blood sugar control and on so many other fronts.

## To Do

- Avoid sugar and processed carbohydrates, such as pasta, bread, pastries, and bagels. Be especially wary of anything made with high-fructose corn syrup.

- Use instead in moderation: raw honey, maple syrup (grade B or C), blackstrap or sorghum molasses, date or palm sugar, stevia, or xylitol.

- Create an exercise program that works for you, after consulting your practitioner.

- Eat a breakfast with high-quality proteins, such as eggs, or a smoothie with whey or rice protein powder and yogurt.

- Keep your life simple and your carbohydrates complex!

- Choose fats that are mostly monounsaturated, such as those from olives and avocados; healthy saturated fats, such as coconut oil; and the omega-3 unsaturated fatty acids found in fish, flaxseeds, and walnuts.

- Feed your cells nutritional superstars, such as chile peppers, buckwheat, and cinnamon.

- Consider supplementing with the mineral chromium (or a good multinutrient containing chromium) to manage and prevent hyperglycemia.

## Last Word

*I found that keeping sugar and sugar-laden products out of my house was the key to keeping them out of my life. It was difficult in the beginning; I had to sit down with my family and explain to them exactly what the stakes were. Once they were on board, it was so much easier. We all agreed to just say no to packaged foods, and made the commitment to make one or two changes every week until I got to where I am today: sugar free, cancer free.*

—Sela S., breast cancer survivor

# CHAPTER 7

# NOURISHING IMMUNITY

*On a planet teeming with microorganisms, the only thing standing between "us" and "them" is the immune system.*

—Dr. Robert Rountree and Carol Colman

> CHAPTER GOAL: Maintain a strong immune system

The immune system is the most diverse system in the body. If you imagine a fortress, then the immune system consists of the walls outside and the soldiers within. The soldiers have a hierarchy of many different functions. Each has a particular job, and yet they interact with one another as a team to effectively defend the fort against invaders like cancer cells.

# Meet Your Immune System

The immune system consists of distinct cellular populations dispatched throughout the body to protect us from invading pathogens, such as viruses, unfriendly bacteria, fungi, and parasites. Immune cells communicate with each other through chemical mediators that regulate and interface with many other bodily systems. The main organs of the immune system include:

- The *bone marrow* (from which all the cells of the mature immune system are initially derived)

- The *thymus*, whose function is to produce mature T cells

- The *spleen*, which serves as our immunologic filter of the blood and is made up of various immune cells (including T cells and NK cells)

- *Lymph nodes*, which are found throughout the body; they house the cells that produce *antibodies*, the proteins that inactivate identifiable foreign trespassers in the body, and they filter the bodily fluid known as *lymph*

There are two fundamental branches of the immune system: innate and adaptive. The *innate*, or *cellular* immune system, attacks any entity considered foreign (like infectious bacteria), and is evolutionarily ancient, literally prereptilian. In other words, it will go after any bacteria, any pathogen, any invader at all.

As we evolved in complexity as mammals, however, we needed something a bit more specialized. The result was the *adaptive* immune system, which recognizes an attacker as potentially harmful and then remembers that pathogen's specific identity so that the body's defense can be better targeted next time and the attackor doesn't have a second chance to inflict a disease state. One such pathogen is the influenza virus, against which we mount a defense using antibodies, or "immune arrows," as immune specialist Dr. Michael Rosenbaum calls them (pers. comm.), to attack and corner the offender.

In a healthy immune system, both branches and all of their cells are well equipped to fight the hordes of invaders (bacteria, viruses, fungi, and parasites) that are looking to set up shop inside us. Because immune cells reproduce so rapidly and some of them have such a short life span (just a few days), our bodies need to invest substantial amounts of energy in keeping the system functioning smoothly. Good nutrition makes this possible. A well-nourished immune system fights off invaders, including cancer, using a coordinated sequence of events.

First, foreign pathogens that invade the body are recognized by specific white blood cells known as *macrophages*, whose responsibilities include scavenging and surveillance. *Dendritic* cells, which are a specialized type of macrophage, identify the invader, and display its name on the dendritic surface, then summon "higher authorities" to help deal with it. These higher authorities are the *lymphocytes*. The first lymphocytes on the scene are called *T-helper cells,* which work to coordinate the overall response. If the pathogen is already known to the immune system, the T-helper cells will likely summon the *cytotoxic T cells* ("*killer T cells*") to help finish off the enemy. If an unknown threat, such as cancer cells, should appear, elite forces known as NK (natural killer) cells are called into action. NK cells, part of our innate immune function, specialize in dealing with new threats. And unlike T cells, they don't need to have had a previous encounter with an invader to go after it; they will attack *anything* that appears to present a danger. For this reason, NK cells are the most active of all of the immune cells when it comes to facing down cancer. Once the immediate threat has passed, *suppressor T cells* do the job of calming the immune system down.

Adequate nourishment for all components of the immune system is essential for ensuring that all of these jobs are carried out with maximum effectiveness. Nutrient insufficiency in the face of a bodily threat inevitably leads to immune weakness, increasing our susceptibility to cancer occurrence or recurrence.

# Factors That Influence Immunity

The immune system responds splendidly to an Eating for Health diet, daily exercise, targeted nutrient support, and inner work, such as prayer and meditation. A battle-fatigued immune system becomes stronger as you provide it with a diverse, whole-food diet that:

- Is rich in unprocessed fruits, vegetables, whole grains, beans, seeds, and nuts

- Is low in poor-quality fats (trans fats, overheated and rancid fats, genetically modified [GM] oils, and highly refined cooking oils) and refined sugars

- Provides lean, hormone- and antibiotic-free protein

- Is abundant in pure water green and herbal teas (we suggest eight 8-ounce glasses of water per day)

## SUGAR WEAKENS IMMUNITY

The food component most damaging to your immune system is refined sugar, which is often referred to as an immunosuppressant. In *Get the Sugar Out: 501 Simple Ways to Cut the Sugar Out of Any Diet*, author Ann Louise Gittleman (2008) warns that no matter what form it takes, sugar paralyzes the immune system in a variety of ways by:

- Hampering the pathogen-killing capability of white blood cells for up to five hours after intake

- Decreasing the manufacture of antibodies

- Hindering the distribution of vitamin C, one of the most critical vitamins for all aspects of immune function

- Creating mineral imbalances and potential allergic effects, both of which dampen immune system functioning

- Countering the action of essential fatty acids, which makes cells more susceptible to invasion by allergens and microbes

Sugar's harmful effects on the immune system were demonstrated in a study (von Känel, Mills, and Dimsdale 2001) that showed a dramatic decrease in several types of immune system cells just two hours after subjects ingested 75 grams of glucose (slightly more than a 20-ounce cola). Keeping in mind that simple carbohydrates break down readily and rapidly into glucose, we can see clearly that the intake of high-glycemic foods has a profound impact on immune response.

## LACK OF SLEEP LOWERS IMMUNE FUNCTION

When we sleep, our bodies refresh and recharge themselves. Sleep and immunity seem inexorably linked. Researchers at the Max Planck Institute for Evolutionary Anthropology report that animals that sleep more show greater resistance to infection; in fact, "evolutionary increases in mammalian sleep durations are strongly associated with an enhancement of immune defences, as measured by the number of immune cells circulating in peripheral blood" (Preston et al. 2009).

The importance of sleep cannot be overstated. In today's 24-7 cycle of endless activity, it's even more important to honor your body with the sleep it requires. Your immune system will thank you.

## EXERCISE ENHANCES IMMUNE FUNCTIONING— TO A POINT

Exercise not only helps your immune system resist infection but also lowers your chances of heart disease, osteoporosis, and cancer. The National Cancer Institute (NCI) (2009) proposes that "physical activity may prevent tumor development by lowering hormone levels, particularly in premenopausal women, lowering levels of insulin and insulin-like growth factor I (IGF-I), improving the immune response, and assisting with weight maintenance to avoid a high body mass and excess body fat." Remember, however, that too much of a good thing is no longer a good thing. Intensive, long-term exercise creates a great deal of free-radical activity, which results in an increase in stress hormones and a decrease in white blood cell activity. Moderation is key!

**Exercise is absolutely essential for your lymph glands.** Exercise is also a great energizer to the lymphatic system, an exquisitely designed network of vessels and nodes (over six hundred) that work throughout your body to normalize fluids, allocate proteins, and scour for toxins.

But unlike the circulatory system, which is outfitted with a dedicated pump (the heart), lymph requires bodily motion to move—another reason to adapt or maintain a regular exercise program! Walking, biking, swimming, rebounding, weight training, running, yoga, and even rhythmically tapping your chest will help stimulate lethargic nodes.

# Evaluating Your Immune Status

A basic complete blood count (CBC) will tell you and your health care practitioner a great deal about your immune system health. Some practitioners may be interested in more subtle tests, for example, lab tests that examine NK cell population and activity (a natural killer cell cytotoxicity assay), and the balance of various cytokines, immune system chemicals that we'll discuss in more depth in the next chapter. But you and your health care provider can also tell much about your immune health by simply observing a history of frequent infection, usually in the upper respiratory tract, or frequent sore throats. Answering yes to any of the following questions is a sign that your immune system needs greater nourishment:

- Do you catch colds easily?
- Do you get more than two colds a year?
- Are you suffering from any chronic infections?
- Do you get frequent cold sores or have recurring genital herpes?
- Are your lymph glands sore and swollen at times?
- Do you now have or have you ever had cancer?

Recurrent or chronic infections, even very mild colds, occur when the immune system is weakened or overwhelmed. Antibiotics can compensate for the work that your immune system has failed to do, but taking antibiotics doesn't replenish the nutrients lost during the battle to rid the body of microbes. Enhancing the immune system with nourishing food and additional nutrients can help break the cycle of immune deficiency and exhaustion.

# Guidelines for Nurturing and Maintaining Immunity

There is much you can do to help foster a healthy immune system. The following are guidelines that you can incorporate into your daily life.

## Slash Your Stress

Along with diet and exercise, stress management is essential to staying well and maintaining a vigilant immune system. Struggling with depression, anxiety, and panic is exhausting to our minds and bodies. Work with a qualified health care provider to examine food sensitivities, nutrient insufficiencies, and drug-nutrient interactions to assess the metabolic effects of unrelenting stress and what you can do about it.

Once you've ruled out or dealt with metabolic issues, try some of the many simple and cost-free techniques to reduce stress and anxiety. Guided imagery involves focusing on mental images, such as a serene setting. Tai chi and some forms of yoga, combining both mental and physical exercise, can help heal mind and body. Consider using biofeedback, a process in which you monitor certain functions of the body, such as blood pressure, and learn to alter these functions through reinforced relaxation. Other simple techniques include deep-breathing exercises or taking a walk and appreciating the beauty in the world around you.

One intriguing study looked at the effects of massage on women who were in active breast cancer treatment. Women diagnosed with breast cancer received either massage therapy three times a week for five weeks or just standard treatment. By the end of the study, the massage-therapy group reported feeling less depressed, less angry, and more energetic. The levels of NK cells also increased from the first to the last day of the study for the massage therapy group (Hernandez-Reif et al. 2005).

## Learn to Love Mushrooms

Many different mushrooms have been studied and consumed for their medicinal properties. Of the many species of mushrooms, holistic medical practitioners most commonly recommend these:

- *Maitake.* Often found at the base of oak trees and esteemed by herbalists all over the world, the maitake mushroom is best known for its ability to stimulate the production of T cells in the blood.

- *Shiitake.* The shiitake mushroom is the most widely recognized medicinal mushroom and is generally used as an immune system booster.

- *Reishi.* Used primarily as a tea or tincture because of its woody texture, this mushroom has been used by the Chinese for thousands of years as an immune system enhancer.

- *Cordyceps.* The extract from the cordyceps mushroom has proven itself to be effective in fighting various forms of bacteria while increasing physical stamina. The sports world took notice of the possible benefits of cordyceps mushrooms in 1993, when nine women who were taking cordyceps reportedly broke world records at the Chinese National Games.

**THE MOUSE SWIM TEST:** One way that the ability of cordyceps to increase energy was measured was through the "mouse swim test," conducted in 1999. In this test, mice were placed in a tank of water and permitted to swim to exhaustion. The mice given cordyceps swam longer than mice that had received a placebo (Holliday and Cleaver 2008).

Recent research has shined a light on mushrooms and their immune-enhancing and anticancer properties. One study of more than 350 women with breast cancer and an equivalent number without it indicated that the women with the highest consumption of mushrooms had a 46 percent lower risk of breast cancer, compared to women with the lowest consumption (Hong et al. 2008). Another team of researchers reported that dietary intake of mushrooms, in combination with green tea, had a dramatic effect on breast cancer risk. Daily consumption of at least 10 grams of fresh mushrooms or at least 4 grams of dried mushrooms was linked to a respective 64 and 47 percent reduction of risk, compared to a diet without mushrooms. The women who both ate mushrooms and drank green tea daily experienced even greater benefits (Zhang et al. 2009).

## What about Whey?

Little Miss Muffet most likely didn't know what she was onto while she was busy eating her curds and whey, the by-products of cheese making. But whey has been shown to be a healthful addition to an anticancer diet, due to its immune-friendly and antioxidant effects.

An excellent source of essential amino acids, whey seems valuable on a number of fronts. For example:

- Whey protein is particularly rich in the amino acid cysteine. Women with high levels of cysteine have a lower rate of breast cancer than women with lower levels of cysteine (Zhang et al. 2003).

- Whey protein concentrate raises glutathione levels substantially. Glutathione is our own internal antioxidant that protects cells and serves as a primary detoxifier of carcinogens and other toxins. Glutathione levels are intimately tied to immune function (Fidelus and Tsan 1986). In fact, whey protein concentrates have been used for years to help improve the immune status of AIDS patients (Micke, Beeh, and Buhl 2002).

- Animals fed whey protein concentrate demonstrated an increased immune response to a variety of pathogens, including salmonella and streptococcus pneumonia (Bounous, Kongshavn, and Gold 1988).

Most whey products today come in the form of a powder that can be added to smoothies for extra protein and immune support.

## THE WHATS OF WHEY

Although whey protein contains considerably less lactose than milk, people with lactose intolerance need to proceed with caution.

Because whey protein is popular with body builders, there are a great variety of whey products on the market. Find a whey product with the words "undenatured" and "cold processed" on the label. This assures you that the most nourishing components of the product have not been over-processed or damaged.

If you put whey in your smoothie, add it just before you stop blending, to preserve its immunoglobulins and other precious nutrients.

# Garlic Is as Good as Ten Mothers

Thus was named a popular 1980 film homage to the wonders of the "stinking rose." But just what is so amazing about garlic? The bountiful bulb is rich in antioxidants that include sulfur-based compounds, flavonoids, and dozens of other health-promoting constituents. These constituents help quench free radicals, and their sulfur content boosts the detoxification powers of the liver. Garlic is also rich in selenium, an essential component of the antioxidant enzyme glutathione peroxidase.

In *Garlic for Health*, Dr. Benjamin Lau (1988) writes, "Garlic apparently stimulates the body's immune system, particularly enhancing the macrophages and lymphocytes, which destroy cancer cells." In 1996, Dr. Herbert Pierson of the U.S. National Cancer Institute noted, "Garlic is a veritable pharmacopeia. That's why garlic has been found in every medical book of every culture ever. For thousands of years, garlic has been used for the treatment and prevention of disease. So there has to be something there" (quoted in Bergner 1996, 1). Need we say more?

## Experiment with Aloe

Hippocrates was the first to write about the virtues of aloe vera, a succulent plant believed to have existed in Africa for thousands of years. Over twenty years ago, N. V. Gribel and V. G. Pashinski (1986) noted that the juice of the aloe vera plant reduced tumor mass and metastases in rats. Interestingly enough, it is the special sugars in the gel of the aloe vera plant that seem to embody the secret of its potency. These sugars are called *glyconutrients*, and unlike simple sugars, such as table sugar, they have no adverse effect on blood sugar. Potent enzymes produced from these glyconutrients appear to boost lymphocyte (a type of white blood cell) production, thus powering up the immune system. What's more, aloe functions as a first-rate antioxidant while protecting the all-important master antioxidant glutathione (Norikura et al. 2002). Aloe vera is available commercially as a juice, gel, or concentrated powder. But why not buy yourself a small aloe plant, scoop a spoonful of gel from inside its prickly leaf, and add it to your smoothie?

## Consider Chlorella

One of your most powerful allies in maintaining healthy immunity is a tiny, single-celled green algae called chlorella. "Chlorella is my favorite whole-food supplement," says Dr. Michael Rosenbaum (pers. comm.), an immune specialist practicing in Corte Madera, California. "It's shown to be a potent immune stimulant, both nourishing and detoxifying. My cancer patients report improved energy, and I see improved white blood cell function in virtually everyone." The reason for this improvement, as Dr. James Balch and Phyllis Balch (1997) explain in *Prescription for Nutritional Healing*, is that chlorella has more chlorophyll per ounce than any other plant. It is made up of almost 58 percent protein and contains carbohydrates, all the B vitamins, vitamins C and E, all nine essential amino acids, enzymes, and rare trace minerals.

Chlorella is available in powder, liquid, or tablet form.

## Glutathione

Few substances can equal the value of glutathione in maintaining overall good health and immune functioning. As the body's most powerful antioxidant and detoxifier, glutathione neutralizes harmful free radicals and eradicates toxins while supporting cellular health and energy. The result is a winning anticancer compound.

Glutathione is composed chiefly of three amino acids—cysteine, glycine, and glutamic acid—and most of our supply is produced in the liver. Without glutathione, our bodies would become overwehelmed with toxins, making it difficult for the immune system to keep up. Glutathione is also used up during stressful episodes, because excessive adrenaline curbs its production.

Eggs, legumes, brassica vegetables (such as broccoli and cabbage), asparagus, avocado, and walnuts are rich dietary sources of glutathione or the compounds the body needs to make glutathione. Glutathione is also available as a *liposomal* cream, a formulation that is thought to enhance absorption and delivery. We'll return to glutathione in chapter 9.

# Your Nutrients for Immunity

As we discussed in chapter 5, certain nutrients exert a profound effect on immune functioning. Recall that vitamins D, C, and A, as well as the carotenoid family (including beta-carotene) and the minerals selenium, zinc, and magnesium, are protectors of immunity and overall cellular health. Chapter 5 lists food sources of these critical nutrients and offers advice on how to choose supplements that contain healthy forms of them.

## Noteworthy Herbs for Immune Balance

Literally hundreds of herbs have been examined for both immune-boosting and cancer-protective properties. While space is limited here, an invaluable resource for learning about herbs and cancer in brilliant detail is herbalist Donald Yance's book *Herbal Medicine, Healing, and Cancer* (1999). According to Yance, the essential beauty of herbs is that they provide a concentrated assortment of phytonutrients that balance and heal injured cells and tissue. They signal the immune system to be more precise in its surveillance and deployment missions. The herbs described next are rich in trace minerals and protective bioflavonoids that send extra healing energy to weary circulating cell defenders.

## ASTRAGALUS

This herb is used for its immune-enhancing properties and to bolster white blood cell counts. In long-established studies from the NCI and other leading U.S. cancer institutes, astragalus has been shown to strengthen the immune system (Sun et. al 1983). Based on these studies, it is evident that astragalus does not attack cancer directly, but instead strengthens the body's immune system.

## CAT'S CLAW (UNO DE GATO)

Cat's claw is a woody vine native to the South American rain forest whose bark has been used traditionally for its immune-enhancing characteristics. While human trials have not yet been conducted, in vitro studies have indicated that alkaloids from the plant intensify the rate of *phagocytosis* (the process of engulfing and destroying foreign particles) and fuel the production of *interleukin*, an important substance produced by white blood cells to help orchestrate incoming attacks on invaders (Lemaire et al. 1999).

## A CAUTIONARY NOTE ABOUT HERBS

Herbs are powerful, complex remedies that contain hundreds of compounds working together synergistically. For this reason, we suggest that you consult with a seasoned herbal practitioner before embarking on a program of herbal supplementation. Be sure to describe your regimen with other practitioners you are seeing, and be alert for potential interactions.

# Bringing It All Together

Dr. Andrew Weil, noted author and director of the Arizona Center for Integrative Medicine at the University of Arizona, has written extensively about the body's ability to heal itself. Consider checking out his book *Natural Health, Natural Medicine: The Complete Guide to Wellness and Self-Care for Optimum Health*, which has a chapter on how to protect your immune health. You can take advantage of the body's innate ability to heal by eating well, exercising regularly, and striving for spiritual well-being. It's important to eliminate negative factors such as drugs, alcohol, tobacco, and other assaults on your body. Smile, play, celebrate, and cherish your precious body.

## TO DO

- Monitor your white blood cell count with a CBC (complete blood count) to make sure you have a healthy population of immune cells.

- Get sufficient sleep and exercise to help maximize immunity, but avoid the tendency to overexercise.

- Practice Eating for Health, especially avoiding sugar, which directly lowers immune function.

- Make sure your diet is rich in selenium, vitamin C, carotenoids, mushrooms, garlic, and other immune-enhancing foods and nutrients.

- Experiment with specialized foods, such as aloe vera, chlorella, and whey protein, to further boost immunity.

- Work with a qualified herbal practitioner to use immune-enhancing herbs effectively and wisely.

- Share your regimen with your other health care practitioners.

## Last Word

*The best part of eating to fortify my immune system was learning to prepare a variety of delicious new foods: mushroom soup, spaghetti squash with pesto sauce, and whey protein bars for midday snacks—yum!*

—Holly G., breast cancer survivor

# CHAPTER 8

# INFLAMMATION

*Wherever flaxseeds become a regular food item among the people, there will be better health.*

—Mahatma Gandhi

> GOAL: Reduce inflammation levels and keep them low

Consider the simple pimple, sunburn, or mosquito bite. Minor ailments such as these produce inflammation. So do worse injuries, like a sprained or broken ankle. But in this chapter, when we talk about inflammation, we are referring to chronic inflammation, the kind you can't feel or know. Experts now believe that chronic inflammation may be linked to various forms of cancer as well as other major diseases, such as rheumatoid arthritis, diabetes, and heart conditions. New studies continually increase our understanding of the complex inflammation process and how it relates to breast cancer. In 2010 several pieces of the inflammation puzzle came together when researchers (Liu et al.) at Thomas Jefferson University definitively demonstrated that breast inflammation is fundamental to the growth and spread of breast cancer.

While the relationship between inflammation levels and breast cancer continues to be closely examined, there are steps you can take to lower chronic inflammation naturally, reduce your risk of recurrence, and improve your overall health at the same time. But first, let's take a closer look at what inflammation is, as well as its causes and effects on the body.

# What Is Inflammation?

Inflammation is your immune system's natural response to an injury, such as a pulled muscle, or to germs, allergens, chemical irritants, and other threats. Your immune system reacts by releasing white blood cells and chemicals into the bloodstream, which infiltrate your tissues, causing the indicators of inflammation that most of us are familiar with: redness, heat, swelling, and pain. There's a biological domino effect at work here: all of these symptoms are created by the activity of immune cells breaking down injured tissue so that fresh, healthy tissue can replace it. This is a normal and appropriate response; our bodies *need* to stay vigilant in order to fend off an invasion or injury with aggressive pro-inflammatory mechanisms, such as clotting, fever, and swelling. But too often, inflammation becomes a chronic condition, and in this state, we leave ourselves more vulnerable to breast cancer occurrence and recurrence.

Here's how: When inflammation arises, chemicals known as inflammatory *cytokines*, or *chemokines* (proteins that serve as messengers between cells) are released into the blood and tissues. These types of cytokines are created primarily by immune cells engaged in the process of mounting an inflammatory response, as a way of dealing with a health threat to the body. By relaying messages between the cells, the cytokines help to modulate the immune system response to whatever threat is at hand. But the presence of too many inflammatory cytokines harms our normal cells—and there's the rub.

# Inflammation and Breast Cancer: An Unwholesome Relationship

We've known for quite some time that inflammation and cancer have shared some sort of functional relationship. In fact, as long ago as 1863, German pathologist Rudolph Virchow first hypothesized that cancer originated at sites of chronic inflammation (Coussens and Werb 2002). Now it seems that modern science has caught up with nineteenth-century observations. It wasn't easy.

It took twelve years and the breeding of a highly specialized mouse for researchers to finally prove that inflammation in the breast is one key to the development of breast cancer (Liu et al. 2010). The researchers in this study specifically tested the activity of a principal inflammatory pathway known as NF-kappaB to assess its effect on breast cancer—no easy task, as the researchers had to find a way to turn off inflammation in the breasts only. And, ingeniously, they did, paving the way to their discovery.

Another noteworthy study (Pierce et al. 2009) confirmed a link between chronic inflammation and breast cancer *recurrence*. In this study, scientists at the Fred Hutchinson Cancer Research Center at the University of Washington noted that women with high levels of two other inflammation markers—*C-reactive protein* and *serum amyloid A*—were more likely to die early or have a cancer recurrence than women with lower levels.

Although many inflammatory substances have been shown to have a relationship with cancer, three of the most widely researched enzymatic compounds to date are known as COX, LOX, and the chemical signal NF-kappaB (and no, Dr. Seuss did not come up with these names!). While the particulars of each enzyme are not critical to this discussion, it is important to understand the need to keep a balance between the "pro-inflammatory" and "anti-inflammatory" forces at work in our bodies.

# Inflammation Enables Angiogenesis

Another important characteristic of chronic inflammation is its relationship to angiogenesis, the development of new blood vessels. COX and LOX are enzymes that promote inflammation, and hormonelike chemicals from these enzymes play a major role in creating new blood vessels. While this is a natural and normal process, it is also one that tumors (even those too small to show up on a mammogram) can hijack to build a blood supply to accommodate their growing needs. Inflammatory cells stimulate the formation of new blood vessels that then transport nutrients and oxygen to the tumor. This is a recipe for chronic inflammation, with each process promoting the other. Clearly, inflammation and the resulting angiogenesis are outcomes that need to be kept under control.

On the flip side, research suggests that enzymes that block inflammation also inhibit angiogenesis, so by inhibiting one of these processes, you are positively affecting both (Jackson et al. 1997).

# Factors That Influence Inflammation

A number of lifestyle factors play a role in contributing to chronic inflammation. Inflammation can be set in motion by your fork and knife. Not surprisingly, packaged foods that are high in sugar or trans fats are among the most potent of pro-inflammatory foods. And the type of fat you eat just might play the biggest role of all in determining levels of systemic inflammation, as you'll see shortly.

## Oxidative Stress

Your body continually combines the oxygen you breathe with nutrients from the food you eat to produce energy. One result is *oxidation*: the stripping of an electron from each atom or molecule the oxygen combines with, creating what biochemists call free radicals (which we've mentioned a number of times previously). Since electrons come in pairs, when molecules lose an electron, they "steal" electrons from other molecules. These molecules then "steal" electrons from other molecules, and so on.

Free-radical activity is a normal part of being alive, and when it is under control, it's part of the engine that drives metabolism. But heavy metals, toxic food, smoking, and all sorts of other internal and external assaults—even an imbalance of nutrients—can rev up this process. This is *oxidative stress*. Unchecked, oxidation can behave like an out-of-control fire, damaging cells, tissues, and organs indiscriminately—the dangerous chain reaction known as *free-radical damage*. In an attempt to repair such damage, the body calls for an immune response, which, in turn, initiates inflammation, and this causes even more free-radical generation. It's a vicious cycle.

One way to keep inflammation and oxidative stress under control is to eat a diet rich in antioxidants. Eight to twelve servings a day of fruits, vegetables, or both should do the trick (see appendix A for tips on incorporating more fruits and veggies into your daily routine).

## Weight and Blood Sugar

Keeping your weight in check is crucial for preventing inflammation, as well as conditions associated with it and obesity, such as heart disease and diabetes. Research indicates that *visceral fat* (the fat located deep in the abdominal area) is more metabolically active than other types of fat, secreting large amounts of inflammatory cytokines (Maury and Brichard 2010). The good news? Maintaining a healthy weight greatly reduces and, in some cases, even eliminates inflammation.

Remember that the hormone insulin, itself, is associated with inflammation (see chapter 6). So, the lower you can keep your fasting glucose and insulin levels, the less you will have to worry about them as a source of unwanted inflammation.

## Stress and Sleep Deprivation

In addition to diet, certain lifestyle choices may contribute to inflammation. According to Dr. Isaac Eliaz (pers. comm.), who practices integrative medicine in Sebastopol, California, both stress and sleep deprivation can lead to inflammation through the elevation of the hormone *cortisol*. Chronic stress, Dr. Eliaz explains, leads to the overproduction of cortisol, the body's most abundant stress hormone. This rise in cortisol disrupts normal hormonal function, raising blood sugar levels and contributing to the inflammatory cascade.

## Excessive Exercise

Everyone feels better with regular exercise. While improving physical fitness and enhancing overall well-being, it may also strengthen the immune system. It's tempting to be impatient and ignore our bodies' protests when we are trying to reach a physical goal, but be careful! When combined with inadequate rest and other stresses, overexercising, sometimes called "overtraining syndrome," can lead to an impaired immune system and inflammation (MacKinnon 2000). One theory as to what causes this chain reaction is that your overtaxed muscles and tissues trigger the release of pro-inflammatory cytokines, the proteins that act as messengers between the cells. When sufficient rest is allowed, pro-inflammatory cytokines facilitate the healing process—but only if rest is allowed. That's why we often feel better if we rest after a long bike ride and why it's best to alternate periods of exercise with periods of healing, recuperative rest.

# Assessing Your Inflammation Status

Other than some obvious signs—puffy gums, sore joints, chronic nasal stuffiness—how can you tell if your inflammation levels are higher than they should be? Several tests can be useful here.

## C-Reactive Protein

*C-reactive protein* (CRP) is a powerful inflammation marker. The pro-duction of CRP is an indispensable part of the inflammation process, and its measurement mirrors the level of inflammation in the body. We believe that measuring inflammation with a high-sensitivity CRP test (HS-CRP), a simple blood test, is one of the most important steps you can take if you have had cancer. If the results are elevated, above 1.0, then it's time to take action to bring down your CRP levels. You might want to retest at three-month intervals. If you don't have cancer but have risk factors, you might consider having the test run on an annual basis as part of your regu-lar physical exam. Some practitioners like to look at other inflammatory markers. A complete inflammatory profile might include, interleukin-1 (IL-1) beta, interleukin-6 (IL-6), interleukin-8 (IL-8), and tumor necrosis factor (TNF).

## Fibrinogen

*Fibrinogen* is a protein produced by the liver that helps the blood to clot properly. Its levels increase in reaction to inflammation, so if inflam-mation levels are high, it may be wise to check fibrinogen levels as well. We recommend that fibrinogen levels range between 215 and 300 milli-grams per deciliter of blood. Bringing levels into normal range has the added benefit of keeping the blood flowing more smoothly, making it more difficult for metastases to develop.

## Food Sensitivity Panel

If your inflammatory markers remain stubbornly high, consider the possibility of food allergies or sensitivities. Common allergens like casein (from dairy) and gluten (from wheat) are known to spark an inflammatory cascade in sensitive individuals. So, one way to cool inflammation on a cellular level is to pay attention to foods that may cause headaches, diges-tive upset, or skin eruptions, like acne or eczema. Keep in mind that as we age, foods that may not have bothered us before, like dairy and wheat, may trigger chronic low-grade inflammation. Even seemingly innocuous foods, when eaten repeatedly, can cause a food sensitivity to develop. If you think you might have a food sensitivity, we recommend going on an elimination diet for two weeks to see how you feel. We deal with the specifics of this later in the chapter. You might also consider doing a food allergy panel through one of the labs listed in appendix B, available through your nutritionist or other holistic practitioner.

## Thermography to Assess Breast Inflammation

Breast thermography provides one of the best visual clues of the presence of inflammation in breast tissue. Since inflammation often accompanies precancerous changes to the breast and since it always produces heat, measuring the temperature of the breasts can provide us with vital information.

Temperature measurement as a means of assessing health has its roots in ancient Greece, when Hippocrates covered his patients' bodies with a thin slurry of mud and, as it dried, observed temperature differences around diseased organs. With the advent of military infrared heat detection technology, specialized cameras were developed that could produce a detailed picture showing how the heat is distributed over the body. This picture could then be analyzed with computer software to determine regions of abnormal heat, suggesting injury or disease.

When it comes to breast health, here's how it works, according to Robert Kane (pers. comm.), a board-certified clinical thermologist who maintains a busy thermal-imaging interpretation practice in Redwood City, California: "Heat is produced in the breast by normal tissue metabolism and is carried to the surface by the blood supply. Our bodies naturally release heat to the environment in the form of infrared energy to maintain a normal body temperature of 98.6 degrees Fahrenheit. This energy can be captured and visualized by a special infrared detector inside the thermography camera."

Normal breast tissue produces a characteristic temperature pattern when visualized with thermography. On the other hand, fast-growing, abnormal breast tissue (cancerous or precancerous) will produce heat through its faster metabolism. This heat travels through the circulatory system to the surface of the skin, where it can be detected using a thermographic camera (Yahara et al. 2003). What's more, as mentioned earlier, cancerous tissue can create its own blood supply via the process of angiogenesis, or new blood vessel formation (Anbar 1994). Both of these occurrences can translate into temperature changes at the surface of the breast and provide a means of detection with the thermographic camera.

Thermography findings are less dependent on the *size* of the abnormal tissue and are more directly related to the degree of inflammation, growth rate of the tissue, and metabolic activity (Gautherie et al. 1982). The more inflamed, aggressive, and metabolically active the tissue, the more likely that a trained interpreter will see it on a thermogram. Since highly inflamed, precancerous growth represents the highest likelihood that cancer will develop, we consider thermography to be an excellent addition to standard breast imaging (mammography, MRI, or ultrasound) to help identify smaller lesions that are growing quickly and may appear between annual examinations.

Perhaps even more important, thermography provides invaluable feedback if you're attempting to lower your risk of recurrence through lifestyle and nutrition, allowing you to see if your actions are effective. In short, just as thermography can be used to identify physiological signs that precede cancer and signal future risk, you can also use it to track the success of your anti-inflammatory strategies, adding a great deal to your peace of mind between conventional screenings.

# Guidelines for Lowering Inflammation

Exactly how does diet influence inflammation? Let us count the ways.

## Change Your Oil

The type of fat that you eat is, quite possibly, the most important dietary factor affecting the level of inflammation in your body. That's because fats are precursors to both pro-inflammatory and anti-inflammatory chemicals. Note that we are *not* saying that *all* fat is bad for you. Fat is as necessary to good health as protein, carbohydrates, and nutrients. But there is a world of difference between healthy fats and unhealthy fats.

**Unhealthy Fats Are Objectionable**

- Fats stimulate a variety of chain reactions in your body. Picture a line of dominoes. When you push on the first one, the rest topple. Inserting unstable or unhealthy fats into the system will eventually cause the system to collapse in the same way, as they initiate a domino effect that ends with a host of pro-inflammatory *eicosinoids* (molecules composed of fatty acids) running rampant.

- When you consider that every cell in your body is surrounded by a lipid (fat) layer that is just the right consistency to let all necessary nutrients *in* while allowing all the critical waste material to pass *out*, you can see that altering the composition of that cell membrane is risky business. Yet, that's exactly what unhealthy fats do. You can think of it like this: they actually gum up your cell membranes, preventing nutrients and wastes from passing in and out as they should.

- Trans fats are among the worst offenders (Mozaffarian et al. 2004). Although they exist nowhere in nature, they line super-market shelves in large quantities in the form of snack foods, fried foods, baked goods, and vegetable shortening. Trans fats also create a wealth of free radicals that damage healthy cells and trigger inflammation. Hundreds of studies have now confirmed the unhealthy link between trans fats and inflammation (see for example, ibid.).

## Don't Believe Everything You Read

According to nutrition educator Mira Dessy, author of the blog *Grains & More* (grainsandmore.blogspot.com), the label on packaged foods doesn't tell the whole story. Loopholes in labeling laws allow manufacturers to list "0 trans fats" if the amount present is less than .5 gram per serving. Keep in mind that a serving size is not the same as a portion size, so you may be getting more trans fats in your snack than you bargained for.

## MIND YOUR EFAS

EFAs, or *essential fatty acids*, are fats that the body can't live without and that we can't synthesize internally and therefore must obtain from food sources. The EFAs we need to survive are known as the omega-6 fatty acids and the omega-3 fatty acids. Simply put, omega-6 fatty acids start the fire of inflammation, and omega-3 fatty acids put it out. Since we need to both start and stop inflammation, we need both types of fat. That's why nature provided us with plenty of both. Most grains, nuts, and seeds contain large amounts of omega-6 fats. These fats work their way up the food chain in several ways. For example, cattle that are fed grass create meat and dairy products that are high in omega-3 fats. These days, cows are fed primarily corn and soy in feedlots, which produces much higher levels of omega-6 fats in the meat and dairy products that result. Because of this and the ubiquitous presence of corn, soy, canola, and other omega-6–rich vegetable oils in processed food and on supermarket shelves, our fat consumption habits have changed dramatically in the last century. Whereas our ancestors are believed to have eaten about twice as many omega-6 fats as omega-3 fats, many experts believe Americans now eat fifteen to seventeen times more omega-6 fats than omega-3 fats (Simopoulos 2006). The result is an unbalanced inflammation response.

An ideal balance of omega-6 to omega-3 fats would go a long way in keeping inflammation under control. Omega-3 fats act as natural COX-2 inhibitors, much like ibuprofen or celecoxib (such as Celebrex), but without the potential side effects. You will want to get your omega-6 fats from whole grains, seeds, and nuts, and to avoid the refined, bleached, and processed oils you find on supermarket shelves (corn, soy, canola, safflower, and so on). And you'll want to incorporate more omega-3 fats into your diet by adding wild salmon, halibut, sardines, and occasional tuna, and by eating lots of flaxseeds, chia seeds, and walnuts, all high in omega-3 fats. Salmon is a particularly rich source of eicosapentaenoic acids and docosahexaenoic acids, the two potent omega-3 fatty acids that are so proficient at extinguishing inflammation. Try to include some oily fish, such as wild Alaskan salmon, in your diet twice a week. If your CRP levels are not where they should be, you might consider adding a fish oil supplement to your regimen, which has proven to be a valuable asset in keeping cancer at bay.

Remember to keep your oils tightly covered in a dark-colored glass bottle. Exposure to air, light, and heat oxidizes oils, rendering them rancid, and rancid oils are potent provocateurs of inflammation.

**What about olive oil?** Olive oil is rich in oleic acid, a member of the family of fatty acids called omega-9, which, although not classified as "essential," provide great anti-inflammatory value. For this reason and all of its other wonderful health benefits, we highly recommend the regular consumption of olive oil. Like other precious oils, be sure to store it in a dark container.

For high-heat cooking and baking, we recommend organic coconut oil, which, although saturated, contains a host of healthy medium-chain triglycerides (MCTs) and other beneficial components.

## Lower Your Glycemic Load

Refined sugar and other foods with high glycemic values elevate insulin levels and put the immune system on high alert. Remember, glycemic load measures the impact of a food on blood sugar levels, and bursts of blood sugar trigger the release of insulin. High insulin levels stimulate the release of pro-inflammatory compounds; what's more, they activate additional enzymes that raise levels of arachidonic acid, another inflammatory compound, in the blood.

A 2005 study from the Harvard School of Public Health found that women who ate high-fiber diets that were rich in fruits, vegetables, and whole grains had lower levels of CRP than women whose diets consisted of primarily refined grains (Esmaillzadeh et al. 2006)—yet another reason to avoid sugar and refined flour products.

## Keep Your Antioxidant Levels High

As we discussed earlier in the chapter, free-radical damage is an unavoidable side effect of being alive. But you mount a strong defense against the oxidative stress and inflammation caused by free radicals by keeping your antioxidant intake high. By eating an Eating for Health diet that's rich in vegetables and fruits, you'll boost your antioxidant capacity in these ways:

- You'll support the main antioxidant enzymes that the body produces internally: glutathione, superoxide dismutase, and catalase.

- You'll get plenty of antioxidant vitamins, minerals, and phyto-nutrients (vitamins A, C, and E; selenium; carotenoids; and bioflavonoids) from the colorful fruits and vegetables, whole grains, nuts, and seeds you eat.

*Resveratrol* is a powerful antioxidant worth trying in supplement form. Produced in plants in response to environmental stressors, this compound has been found in dozens of plant species but appears most prominently in the skins of red grapes. Scientists have noted that it exerts a variety of anticancer effects, among them the inhibition of NF-kappaB, one of the harmful inflammatory compounds mentioned earlier (Gao et al. 2001). Bill Sardi (2007), resveratrol expert and author of *You Don't Have to Be Afraid of Cancer Anymore*, recommends 30 to 50 milligrams as a preventative dose, and 300 milligrams or higher for those with an active tumor.

## Don't Forget These Key Nutrients

Be sure to include the following important nutrients in your diet.

### MAGNESIUM

Magnesium is good for so many things, and inflammation is no exception. Researchers who examined data from the National Health and Nutrition Examination Survey (NHANES) 1999–2000, a US national survey, found that American adults who consumed less than the RDA of magnesium (approximately 320 milligrams per day) were 1.48 to 1.75 times more likely to have elevated CRP levels than those who consumed at least the RDA (King et al. 2006). This same survey found that 68 percent of the population surveyed consumed less than the RDA of magnesium. Remember your food sources of magnesium: whole grains (especially buckwheat and oats), nuts, beans, artichokes, and most green, leafy vegetables.

## VITAMIN D

In chapter 5 we discussed how vitamin D can help enhance immunity and cell differentiation. It turns out it can do a lot more than that. Another significant marker of inflammation, known as serum TNF-α, appears to go up as vitamin D levels go down (Petersen and Heffernan 2008). This may help explain the role of this vitamin in the prevention and treatment of other inflammatory diseases, including heart disease, multiple sclerosis, and rheumatoid arthritis.

# *Monitor Food Allergies and Sensitivities*

Any time you eat a food to which your body is allergic or sensitive, your body views the food as a foreign invader and mounts an immune and inflammatory response. There are many labs that will test you for food allergies and sensitivities (see appendix B), but you can also test yourself without too much fuss. Here's how to do it.

## ELIMINATION DIET

An elimination diet, described by Dr. William Crook in 1988, removes the most highly allergenic foods from the diet in an effort to allow your body to recover from any symptoms that may be caused by sensitivity to these foods. Sensitivity issues can include bloating, diarrhea, constipation, itching, mental fogginess, and cravings for a particular food. We encourage people to use a food log during this period to ensure the notation of any symptoms, their cessation, and their possible return. The foods typically removed from the diet are dairy, eggs, gluten (wheat, barley, rye, and spelt), soy, corn, red meat, peanuts, all other nuts, citrus, and shellfish. These foods are avoided for approximately twenty-one days. At the end of this period, foods are added back in one at a time every three to five days, while the return of any symptoms is noted.

## ROTATION DIET

Rotation diets allow people to moderate how often they eat certain foods, with the aim of avoiding potential allergic or sensitivity responses caused by eating certain foods too often. By rotating how often you eat foods to which you may have a low-level sensitivity, you can reduce your exposure and your symptoms. This diet also allows you to clearly identify which foods you are reacting to, since you are eating them only every four to five days. In our experience, following a rotation diet can allow the immune system to repair itself through the avoidance of cumulative exposure.

## Spice Up Your Life

A wholesome dose of curry may do more than add spice to your life. Although curry has been used extensively in Eastern cuisine and has been a staple of Ayurvedic medicine for centuries, we now recognize the active ingredient in it that is responsible for its potent antioxidant and anti-inflammatory effects: *curcumin*.

Research in the last fifty years has repeatedly shown the ability of curcumin to suppress the COX-2 and LOX enzymes and to inhibit metastasis, or tumor spread (Aggarwal et al. 2006). For example, in a mouse study of breast cancer, 68 percent of the mice that received curcumin showed no or very few lung metastases. Among the animals that did not receive curcumin, 83 percent showed extensive metastases (Bachmeier et al. 2007).

Curcumin has shown such power as an anti-inflammatory, anti-metastatic, and apoptosis-inducing agent that it has been the subject of several clinical trials at MD Anderson Cancer Center (see, for example, Aggarwal et al. 2005). Not bad for a kitchen spice!

Boswellia, a powerful herb known as frankincense to our ancestors, is a premier natural LOX inhibitor. And ginger, yet another powerful LOX inhibitor, is also useful in lowering levels of the inflammatory substance PGE2 (Grzanna, Lindmark, and Frondoza 2005). Its power as an antioxidant adds yet another credential to its portfolio of anticancer activity.

While space restricts us from providing a detailed explanation of all the herbs and spices that can offset inflammation, there are dozens, if not hundreds, of botanical compounds that do exactly that. Use the following chart as a starting place to help you remember what to pick at the grocery, the farmers market, or, ideally, your own garden.

## TABLE 8.1 A FEW SUGGESTED
## ANTI-INFLAMMATORY HERBS AND SPICES

| | | | |
|---|---|---|---|
| Basil | Cinnamon | Nutmeg | Sage |
| Bay leaves | Garlic | Oregano | Stinging nettles |
| Boswellia (Frankincense) | Mint | Parsley | Thyme |
| | Mustard | Rosemary | Tulsi (Holy Basil) |
| Cayenne | | | |

**Note:** Herbs can exert a variety of effects. Although generally regarded as safe, some herbs are contraindicated in pregnancy, some may cause allergic reactions in sensitive individuals, and others may need to be avoided due to interactions with pharmaceutical medications. Be sure to check with a knowledgeable practitioner before loading up on herbal supplements.

# Exercise

While activity throughout your lifetime is important, activity at any age can help lower breast-cancer risk. Exercise does more than help you maintain a healthy weight: a 2002 study from the Emory University School of Medicine (Abramson and Vaccarino) found that people aged forty and older who exercised four to twenty-one times a month also experienced decreased levels of CRP.

# Bringing Down Elevated Fibrinogen

Omega-3 oils found in flaxseeds and chia seeds, walnuts, salmon, anchovies, and halibut will not only help to lower elevated CRP levels, but also exert a mildly thinning effect on the blood by bringing down elevated fibrinogen levels. Since "thicker" blood helps cancer to proliferate, some former cancer patients also use *nattokinase*, an enzyme extracted from a fermented Asian soy dish called *natto*, to keep fibrinogen levels at a moderate level. Garlic, vitamin C, and the enzyme bromelain are also helpful in this regard.

125

## TO DO

- Monitor your levels of inflammation by asking your doctor to check your blood levels of C-reactive protein and fibrinogen. Thermography is also available in some communities to examine inflammation patterns in the breasts.

- Change your oil to keep inflammation levels under control. Choose monounsaturated oils such as olive oil (extra virgin) for cold or low-heat use, and coconut oil for higher-heat use. Avoid omega-6 "supermarket" oils, especially the "big four" that are genetically modified: corn, soy, canola, and cottonseed. Eat wild fatty fish, take a fish oil supplement regularly, or do both.

- Follow the recommendations in chapter 6 to keep glucose and insulin levels under control, because high levels of either promote inflammation.

- Be alert for food allergies and sensitivities as a possible cause of systemic inflammation, and test for them if you are suspicious.

- Use culinary herbs and spices liberally in your cooking, because virtually all herbs and spices have anti-inflammatory effects, particularly turmeric, ginger, and boswellia.

- Get sufficient rest and exercise in moderation.

## Last Word

*Eating for inflammation control is really just Eating for Health with a little extra fish oil thrown in. Easy!*

—Michelle B., breast cancer survivor

# CHAPTER 9

# THE KEYS TO LOWERING YOUR TOXIC BURDEN

*Is life worth living? It all depends on the liver.*

—William James

> CHAPTER GOAL: Promote healthy digestion, elimination, and detoxification—keys to cancer prevention

We're all familiar with the phrase, "You are what you eat." We might embellish it a bit by saying, "You are what you assimilate and are unable to eliminate." In essence, we can absorb essential nutrients and eliminate toxins and carcinogens only if we possess vigorous gut and liver health. And although none of us is exempt from the consequences of faulty digestion and elimination, we can all take steps toward improving these bodily functions. In this way, we lower our cancer risk and improve our general well-being.

That's where we'll put our focus in this chapter.

# Meet Your Second Brain

Your digestive system constantly works to break down food to release nutrients that nourish and energize your body. Digestion is controlled by the *autonomic nervous system* (ANS), the part of the nervous system that controls our involuntary bodily functions and acts as the main switchboard for signaling each phase of the digestive process. For the digestive system to work properly, the ANS and the digestive system must "dance" the digestion cha-cha-cha.

## When the Digestion Cha-Cha-Cha Is Blah-Blah-Blah

The big picture is that the intestinal tract, once considered merely a conduit for the transport of food and nutrients, is a complex organism unto itself. An integral part of the body's neuro-endo-immune system, it responds to both internal stimuli and stimuli from the environment. For example:

- It is estimated that over 60 percent of the immune system is located in the intestinal tract (Lipski 2005).

- Because of the intimate association between the gut and the brain, eating under stress constricts bowel function and diminishes immune activity. This is particularly unhealthy because being constipated can cause us to reabsorb bowel toxins (Gershon 1998).

- Incomplete chewing of your food places an unnecessary burden on your entire digestive system and can lead to systemic inflammation.

- Contrary to popular opinion, it's actually a *lack* of stomach acid that causes heartburn and other upper GI symptoms for many people.

- The integrity of the intestinal wall must be intact for proper absorption of nutrients to occur. If the intestinal wall is too porous (from infection, stress, drugs, or toxins, such as chlorine), large protein fragments will get through it and go right into the bloodstream, setting the body up for allergies and inflammation.

- In our practices, we have noticed that about half of our clients over sixty years old do not produce sufficient stomach acid to adequately process their food. We've also observed that a minimum of 30 percent of our clients have an imbalance of yeast, harmful bacteria, or other pathogens inhabiting their intestines.

- Due to a number of factors, including using antibiotics and drinking chlorinated water, most of us are deficient in healthy bacteria. These beneficial microorganisms not only help protect us from pathogens (unfriendly microorganisms) but also manufacture vitamin K and some of the B vitamins. And, they help us eliminate excess estrogen.

As you can see, anything that compromises digestion can have a profound effect on the health and equilibrium of your entire body. Let's take

a closer look at some ways to lose the digestive blahs and keep your digestion dancing, thus maximizing your ability to keep breast cancer at bay.

# Assessing Your General Digestive Status

Indications of poor digestion manifest in various ways, sometimes as symptoms that seemingly have nothing to do with your gut. Here are just *some*
of the signs to pay attention to (Lipski 2005):

| | |
|---|---|
| Abdominal pain | Iron deficiency |
| Bloating | Asthma |
| Constipation | Joint pain or arthritis |
| Diarrhea | Skin conditions, such as eczema, psoriasis, acne, or rosacea |
| Rectal itching | |
| Undigested food particles in stool | Fuzzy thinking and poor memory |
| Poor immunity | Chronic autoimmune disorders |
| Recurrent vaginal infections | |

## Lab Assessments

To get a clearer picture of *exactly* what's going on in your gut, you can
get a stool panel analysis by a lab such as DiagnosTechs or Metametrix.
Simply order this panel through a doctor, nutritionist, or other qualified
health care provider who is familiar with their use. This test offers unique
insights into what is happening in your gut from a *functional* perspective:
Do you have an overgrowth of yeast or other pathogens plaguing your
small intestine? How robust is your supply of friendly microbes? Are you
producing sufficient stomach acid and pancreatic enzymes to adequately
digest your food? How healthy is your gut lining? Stool tests that look at
these indicators can also help determine sensitivities and allergies to

common dietary irritants, such as wheat, dairy, and soy. The great value of these tests lies in their ability to help you and your practitioner pinpoint your digestive problems to find more targeted solutions. And since so many health issues begin in the gut, by repairing it, you are contributing manifestly to your overall well-being.

# Guidelines for Maintaining Healthy Digestion

Once you've got a clearer sense of what may be getting in the way of optimal digestion, absorption, or assimilation, you're ready to go to work. Remember, keeping your inner ecosystem clean is key to preventing cancer from rearing its head.

## Keep Things Moving

As with any complex system, your body needs to get rid of its waste on a regular basis, from one to three times a day. Less-frequent evacuation "backs up the tank," leaving excess toxins behind. Remember, when it comes to helping keep cancer at bay, staying free of toxins is key.

So what does a "perfect" stool look like? Think "The Story of the Three Bears," featuring Goldilocks: not too soft, not too hard; not too pale, not too dark. Eating a varied Eating for Health diet, with plenty of fiber, should keep things running smoothly. If your bowels still move more slowly than you'd like, try adding an additional 500 to 1,000 milligrams of magnesium, a natural laxative, to your daily regimen.

## Get to Know the Bugs in Your Belly

As adults, we all have three to four pounds of bacteria and yeast living within our intestines. This translates to hundreds of trillions of intestinal bacteria, a number that many experts consider to be almost ten times the number of cells in the entire human body (see, for example, Lipski 2005). In a healthy person, more than four hundred species of beneficial organisms flourish in the intestinal tract, aiding in digestion and in the production of B vitamins, vitamin K, and numerous enzymes (Guarner and Malagelada 2003). When health-eroding, pathogenic bacteria get the upper hand, however, we experience digestive distress, impaired detoxification, and increased risk for all diseases, including breast cancer. Your goal is to make sure the beneficial bacteria in your gut far outnumber the pathogenic freeloaders.

## MASTERFUL MICROBES: YOUR VERY BEST FRIENDS

The term *probiotic*, a compound of Latin and Greek words meaning "favorable to life," is popularly used to refer to the helpful bacteria that populate your gut (while technically the term refers to a supplement of these beneficial bacteria). Our ancestors appear to have been well aware of the connection between beneficial bacteria and good health, as we consider the number of age-old fermented foods, rich in healthful bacteria, such as yogurt, sauerkraut, and kimchi, that nourished generations worldwide for centuries.

But every time you take an antibiotic or drink large amounts of chlorinated tap water, you kill off billions of these naturally occurring beneficial bacteria, upsetting the intricate balance of your intestinal terrain. Opportunistic organisms, such as yeast and hostile bacteria, can then flourish, creating a state of imbalance known as *dysbiosis*. The most common type of opportunistic yeast, *Candida albicans*, is a glutton for sugar, which often results in cravings for carbohydrates, such as sugar, pasta, and bread. Prescription antibiotics also modify the natural environment of your intestines; what's more, the abundance of antibiotics in the meats and other commercial animal products we consume *also* contribute to this intestinal imbalance. This makes the choice of organic, grass-fed, antibiotic-free animal products all the more vital.

## GUT FLORA AND ESTROGEN

Recent research has shed intriguing light on the cancer-protective connection between maintaining healthy estrogen levels and healthy gut flora (Boccardo et al. 2006), especially when you consume generous amounts of lignans. *Lignans* are a group of phytonutrients found in seeds, legumes, grains, and vegetables. Flaxseed is by far the richest source of plant lignans, found in the fibrous hull of the seed. Researchers first noted the beneficial activity of flax lignans in the 1980s, when they reported lower levels of lignans in breast-cancer patients than in cancer-free women (Adlercreutz et al. 1986). While the puzzle pieces have not been entirely put together, we do know that when we eat plant lignans, intestinal bacteria convert them into *enterolactones* and *enterodiol*, compounds believed to lower estrogen levels and exert anticancer effects.

## AN OUNCE OF PROBIOTICS: A POUND OF CURE?

Making sure you have plenty of healthy bacteria in your gut is a wise investment. If you enjoy fresh yogurt or other fermented foods, you're already ahead of the game. If not, check out Sally Fallon's *Nourishing Traditions: The Cookbook That Challenges Politically Correct Nutrition and the Diet Dictocrats*, or Sandor Katz's *Wild Fermentation: The Flavor, Nutrition, and Craft of Live-Culture Foods*, two excellent books with step-by-step instructions for transforming your diet into a probiotic powerhouse. An alternative is to take a probiotic supplement daily. Look for one with several different strains of bacteria, such as *L. acidophilus, L. bulgaricus, L. brevis*, and *B. bifidum*. (For a complete list, see *Digestive Wellness*, by Elizabeth Lipski [2005].) If you must take an antibiotic, a course of *saccharomyces boulardii*, a special probiotic yeast supplement sometimes known as "yeast against yeast," taken along with the antibiotic therapy will help restore equilibrium in your gut, protecting it from the *unhealthy* form of yeast (*Candida albicans*) that commonly plagues people who take antibiotics.

## *Plugging the Leaks in Leaky Gut*

The intestinal tract is lined with cells designed to allow well-digested food to pass through it and to serve as a barrier to pathogens, other undesirable substances, and particles too large to benefit our well-being. Stress, pharmaceuticals, and toxins can slowly wear down this protective barrier, creating a condition called *leaky gut*. Leaky gut leaves a gateway through which undesirable substances can enter the body. This, in turn, can stimulate the immune system to respond in the form of allergies, inflammation, and autoimmune conditions. The longer the leaky gut persists, the longer our intestines "lay out the welcome mat" to both external and internal contaminants. A stool analysis will provide an indication of the state of your gut lining, but your holistic practitioner may also recommend an assessment known as an *intestinal permeability test*. Once it is determined that leaky gut is an issue, there are several steps you can take. The ones that we have found to be successful in our practices include:

- Consuming a varied diet of Eating for Health foods to avoid toxicity and to help keep your intestines at an ideal pH for optimal digestive health.

- Emphasizing fermented foods, which provide healthy bacteria, and fresh fruits and vegetables, which provide just the right *prebiotic* nourishment for healthy bacteria (prebiotics are food ingredients, often fiber, that feed intestinal bacteria).

- Avoiding alcoholic beverages, which can interfere with efficient detoxification and put additional strain on the digestive tract.

- Using antibiotics only when absolutely necessary, and carefully heeding the precautions detailed previously.

- Using nonsteroidal anti-inflammatory medications (NSAIDs) sparingly, if at all, because they can erode your delicate gut lining.

- Using a water filter to eliminate chlorine and chloramines from treated tap water.

- Looking out for symptoms associated with common food allergens, such as headaches, bloating, skin eruptions, and brain fog. Ask your practitioner about food-allergy testing if you suspect a problem.

- Taking herbs such as chamomile, yarrow, kudzu, slippery elm, and marshmallow root, and the amino acid L-glutamine to normalize and heal gut mucosa.

- Scheduling relaxation into your life in the same way that you schedule exercise. Putting time aside daily will yield huge rewards.

# When the Staff of Life Becomes the Stuff of Strife

Gluten intolerance is on the rise. Celiac disease, the most serious form of gluten intolerance, is thought to affect approximately 1 percent of the population, a staggering number in absolute terms and far larger than thought just a decade ago (Fasano et al. 2003). The number of people with some level of sensitivity to gluten in the United States may easily run into the tens of millions. Undiagnosed gluten intolerance or even a mild sensitivity strains your entire system by instigating intestinal and then systemic inflammation. For this reason we encourage you to be aware of whether you are gluten sensitive, and we counsel everyone to keep their gluten intake low. Wheat is by far the most glutenous grain, but barley and rye also contain plenty of gluten. A thorough discussion of the potential problems with gluten is beyond the scope of this book, but in the following table we provide some helpful alternatives to glutenous grains and some tips on how to use them in cooking and baking.

| Product | Use |
| --- | --- |
| Amaranth | Use with other flours, because it gets dry and sticky if used alone. Provides complete protein and is rich in minerals. Has more calcium than milk. |
| Brown rice | Wonderful side dish. Also great for breads, muffins, and cookies where a bran taste is desired. High in nutrients. |
| Buckwheat | Groats make a wonderful side dish. Contains gluten analogue that is well tolerated by gluten-sensitive people. Use flour alone as a base for gluten-free cake. |
| Corn flour | Blend with cornmeal or other nonglutenous flours for corn bread, corn muffins, or corn pancakes. |

| Millet | Tasty side dish. Considered one of the least allergenic and most easily digested of all grains. High in protein and minerals. Rich in lecithin. |
| --- | --- |
| Potato flour | Heavy flour with a definite potato taste. Do not confuse with potato starch, a good thickening agent. |
| Oat flour | Adds moist sweetness to baked goods when combined with other flours. Well tolerated by most gluten-sensitive people but may affect a small minority. |
| Quinoa | Strong flavor. Complete protein. Makes a wonderful side dish and works well in cake recipes as a flour. |

# Maximizing Your Digestive Power

By age forty-five or fifty, many of us have stopped producing hydrochloric acid (HCl), the stomach acid we need to thoroughly digest our food. Pancreatic function may have slowed down as well, resulting in less-than-optimal levels of digestive enzymes. These deficiencies often manifest as bloating and other bothersome symptoms, although many people exhibit symptoms that are more subtle and not as clearly related (such as iron-deficiency anemia or weak fingernails). Whether these deficiencies are recognized symptomatically or systematically via medical tests, we suggest taking immediate steps to correct them. For a deficiency of hydrochloric acid (HCl), we recommend the following:

- Take bitter herbs, such as Swedish bitters or a gentian tincture, twenty minutes prior to eating.

- With each meal, drink one teaspoon of apple cider vinegar mixed with warm water, as suggested by Dr. D. C. Jarvis (1958) in his classic book *Folk Medicine: A Vermont Doctor's Guide to Good Health*, to improve digestion and help with a variety of conditions, including balancing pH. Dr. Jarvis suggests using one teaspoon of honey with each teaspoon of cider vinegar if the vinegar alone is too sour. In most cases, people can tolerate up to 3 teaspoons of each. If you experience any burning sensations anywhere along the digestive tract, it's best to stop taking vinegar or to neutralize the discomfort by taking baking soda in water or drinking a small glass of milk.

- Take an HCl supplement, available at your health food store or through your health practitioner. The amount of HCl a person needs can vary from 30 to 100 grains. Start with one capsule per meal and build to tolerance. A burning sensation in the stomach will tell you that you have taken too much.

Once your HCl is back in check, your pancreatic enzymes should follow suit, since HCl signals the release of these enzymes. However, if you are still symptomatic or continue to test low in HCl, add a pancreatic enzyme supplement at the beginning of each meal. We strongly suggest working with a nutrition consultant or other qualified practitioner to assess your status and to determine the best remedies.

## "Nature Will Castigate Those Who Don't Masticate"

Horace Fletcher (1849–1919), also known as "The Great Masticator," coined this phrase as part of a Victorian-era campaign to get people to chew their food more vigorously. Fletcher maintained that people should chew their food about thirty-two times before swallowing it. The eccentric masticator and his adherents took it to the limit, even arguing that liquids, too, had to be chewed in order to correctly mix with saliva.

While we certainly don't advocate chewing your vegetable broth, we're sympathetic to Fletcher's basic premise: chewing your food thoroughly may be one of the most important habits you can cultivate to improve your digestion. Chewing thoroughly helps all the other players on your digestive team do their best work. And as a bonus, your food will taste better!

## The Importance of Loving Your Liver

The largest organ in the body, the liver weighs three to four pounds. It's a complex chemical factory and master orchestrator of bodily functions that works twenty-four hours a day. All the blood that circulates throughout the body to and from the heart passes through the liver. This means that every calorie, nutrient, and chemical we digest passes through the liver for a round of enzymatic activity before being absorbed into the bloodstream.

The protective role of the liver makes it an organ of utmost importance. The liver plays a crucial role in helping the body to break down nutrients and to build new tissues, while it serves as a storage depot for several essential nutrients, such as vitamins A and D, and the minerals iron and copper. The liver is also the body's mastermind when it comes to detoxifying, or getting rid of foreign substances or toxins, whether they come from outside the body (pollutants, plastics, pesticides, and so on) or from metabolic by-products inside it (aggressive estrogens [see chapter 10] and by-products from intestinal bacteria).

## Your Liver Does the "Two-Step"

Using a two-step process, a healthy liver mobilizes an army of specialized enzymes designed to neutralize harmful substances, food additives, and pharmaceutical drugs. In what's commonly known as phase I of the process, the liver neutralizes offending compounds immediately. But if they are fat soluble (that is, they dissolve in fats or oils, not water), the liver must convert them to a water-soluble form first so that they can be excreted in urine or in *bile*, which carries toxins from the liver to the intestines. This second step is known as phase II. The liver generally uses whatever route is needed to rid the body of the chemical as quickly and safely as possible. That's why it's so vital that both phases of the detoxification process coordinate and run smoothly.

## Compromised Detoxification and Cancer Promotion

A well-functioning liver is an essential component of your breast-cancer prevention program, because the liver is a fundamental part of your body's natural filtration system. The activity of your liver's detoxification enzymes is unique, based on your genetics, your level of toxic exposures, and your nutritional status. A well-cared-for liver will function to clear excess estrogens from the body, particularly those that can be carcino-genic. (For a more complete explanation, see chapter 10). The more nutri-tional support you give your liver, the less damage it will take on as it works to keep your body free of carcinogens.

The most important antioxidant for neutralizing toxins produced in phase I is glutathione, sometimes known as the "master antioxidant." Our bodies synthesize glutathione from three amino acids: glycine, cysteine, and glutamate. If our bodies cannot make enough glutathione to keep up with the toxic load from infections and toxins, we can damage the liver, cause immune dysfunction, or both. Stress can also deplete glutathione, because increased adrenaline suppresses its production (Michelle Alpert, DO, pers. comm.).

Vitamin E and selenium are important precursors to glutathione activ-ity, as well as powerful antioxidants in their own right. Although glutathi-one is poorly absorbed as an oral supplement, some doctors offer it as an intravenous drip in their offices, while specialized supplement companies sell liposomal glutathione creams that are reputed to have far better absorption rates. We've seen better results with these liposomal forms.

## SOME PRECAUTIONS CONCERNING DETOXIFICATION

Grapefruit juice and certain pharmaceuticals can have a potent effect on both phase I and phase II detoxification tasks. Grapefruit juice, which contains the phytonutrient naringenin, slows down phase I enzyme activ-ity, making the effect of many medications stronger. For this reason, we suggest that you *not* eat more than half a grapefruit or 4 ounces of grape-fruit juice per day if you are on medication. In addition, do not eat grape-fruit near the time that you take the medication. Medications such as acetaminophen (for example, Tylenol) interfere with phase II activities and, when combined with alcohol, can be highly toxic to the liver.

# Assessing Your Liver Status

Your health care practitioner can tell a great deal about your liver health by looking at some basic blood work. For example, if your liver cells have been damaged by disease, alcohol, or other toxins, levels of certain enzymes in your blood will be high.

What your blood work *won't* tell you is exactly how well your liver is carrying out its detoxification duties. A *comprehensive metabolic profile test* (CMP) that measures all the by-products of your liver's several detoxification "pathways" can give you and your health care practitioner a better idea of exactly how well your liver is functioning (see appendix B for details).

# 50 (or So) Ways to Love Your Liver

Vitamins and minerals, especially the B vitamins, play starring roles in activating the enzymes involved in liver detoxification. Healthy whole grains supply plentiful amounts of B vitamins, which assist the liver with its many detoxification tasks.

We can shore up our liver health by eating clean food and by drinking plenty of nourishing beverages, such as purified water, herbal teas, green tea, fresh juices, and mineral broths found on the Eating for Health food model. Excessive coffee, black tea, soft drinks, diet drinks, sport drinks, and alcohol, especially when combined with environmental chemicals and medications, can harm the liver and interfere with its ability to function.

Support the health of your liver by eating green, yellow, orange, and purple foods from plant sources. Antioxidant vitamins and minerals, such as vitamins A, C, and E; zinc; and selenium are also very helpful. And, the sulfur found in eggs, broccoli, and cabbage—along with the amino acids glycine, cysteine, and glutamine mentioned earlier—help the liver make glutathione.

## "When Life Gives You a Lemon…

…squeeze it, mix it with 6 ounces of distilled water, and drink twice daily," quipped Ann Heustad, RN, in a 2004 newspaper column. Lemon juice helps stimulate the cleansing action of the liver. Although lemon tastes acidic, it helps raise the pH of your saliva, making it more alkaline. This helps you better absorb your nutrients.

Try the juice of half a lemon in a glass of water when you wake up, for a powerful, cleansing way to start the day. Or mix lemon with olive oil in the evening for a potent liver and gallbladder flush while you sleep. Don't undervalue the effectiveness of this underappreciated fruit.

Oranges and tangerines are also powerful liver-supportive fruits, because they, too, contain *limonene*, a phytochemical that has been found to thwart cancer in animal models (Patil et al. 2009). The protective characteristics of limonene are likely due to the fact that it is a strong stimulator of both phase I and phase II detoxification enzymes.

## Fiber Packs a Punch—Again

Every day, the liver produces about a quart of bile, which transports toxins to be dumped into the intestines. Once inside the intestines, the bile, with its toxic cargo, gets absorbed by fiber and is eliminated. A diet low in fiber will undermine this process, so please recall that the Eating for Health model recommends 30 to 40 grams of fiber daily.

## Beets

Beets improve liver function primarily by thinning the bile so that it can move more freely through the liver and into the small intestine. There, it breaks down fat and fuels peristalsis, helping to efficiently move waste out of the body. Look for organically grown beets, because as a root crop, beets are notoriously prone to absorbing toxins in the soil. We like to roast beets in the oven in pieces, covered with a thin layer of olive oil and thickly sliced organic onions.

## Onions and Garlic

We already know that onions and garlic are tasty complements to some of our favorite dishes, but they have proven medicinal, liver cleansing qualities as well. In recent years, researchers have found that the benefits of these vegetables extend to cancer prevention as well. The NCI administered a variety of studies attesting to this fact and even published a fact sheet called *Garlic and Cancer Prevention* (Thomas 2010), in which it asserts, "A host of studies provide compelling evidence that garlic and its organic allyl sulfur components are effective inhibitors of the cancer process." What's more, "These studies reveal that the benefits of garlic are not limited to a specific species, to a particular tissue, or to a specific carcinogen." Could this be part of the secret sauce that makes adherents of the Mediterranean diet so healthful? We suspect so!

Other foods containing liver-cleansing factors include eggs, which, like onions and garlic, are high in sulfur; high-fiber foods, such as apples, celery, legumes, oat bran, and pears; brassica vegetables, such as bok choy, broccoli, and Brussels sprouts; and the spices cinnamon, licorice, and turmeric.

## Liver-Loving Herbs

Used in various civilizations for over two thousand years as a therapy for liver and gallbladder problems, milk thistle is probably the herb most recognized in association with liver health. Milk thistle seems to help the liver in three distinct ways: First, it appears to help the liver regenerate via its antioxidant and anti-inflammatory properties (Song et al. 2006). Second, the active ingredient, silymarin, can help prevent the uptake of toxins into the cells. And third, milk thistle actually helps repair damaged liver cells. In other words, milk thistle may have direct anticancer properties by virtue of its anti-inflammatory, antimetastatic, and regulatory effects on the cancer cell cycle (Ramasamy and Agarwal 2008).

Along with milk thistle, the herbs yellow dock, Oregon grape root, dandelion, Schisandra, and orange peel have also long been associated with liver vitality.

Before using herbs medicinally, always check with a competent herbalist or other qualified practitioner for possible interactions with medications and other herbs or supplements you may be taking.

# Another Word about Exercise

Along with its other virtues, exercise benefits the liver, because it gets the blood and lymph circulating, promoting detoxification. As we mentioned in chapter 7, the movement of lymph relies completely on muscle contraction through physical exercise. Without sufficient lymphatic circulation, cells are left to fester in their own waste. This may contribute to not only cancer but also arthritis and other degenerative diseases, as well as the aging process itself. Aerobic exercise increases lymphatic flow, which means that the body can eliminate more toxins with regular aerobic exercise. The very best way to do this is by jumping rope or bouncing on a mini trampoline, but any aerobic exercise is useful.

Keep in mind, however, that restrictive clothing inhibits the flow of both lymph and blood. Underwire bras and sports bras particularly tend to thwart normal lymphatic flow. If possible, take off your bra while walking and doing other exercise. Doing so will lightly massage the breasts by helping to pump the lymph through the breast tissue.

## To Do

- Increase your lignan intake by adding seeds (especially flaxseeds), legumes, grains, and vegetables to your diet.

- Make sure you are getting a healthy dose of friendly bacteria, either through fermented foods or via a multistrain, well-balanced probiotic supplement.

- Assess your digestive status with the help of a professional to see if you need supportive enzymes or extra hydrochloric acid.

- Be mindful of your bowel health and eat a diet high in fiber and whole foods, supplementing with magnesium, if necessary, to keep things moving.

- Eat plenty of sulfur-rich foods, such as cruciferous vegetables and garlic, daily to keep your liver's detoxification process in top form.

- Drink the juice of half a lemon in 6 ounces of water every morning as a good detoxifying start to your day.

- Consider the liver-loving herb milk thistle, due to its liver-protective *and* cancer-protective effects.

- Exercise regularly to enhance lymphatic flow. Jumping on a mini trampoline, or rebounder, is a wonderful choice for this.

- Limit your use of sports bras and underwire bras to when you feel they are absolutely necessary.

## Last Word

*Cleansing and detoxifying are things I never thought about until after my diagnosis. Now they're a part of my everyday life. I started by adding more water and tea; I used to just drink coffee in the morning and a soda or two after that. Now I drink six to eight cups of hot water with lemon or herb tea (or both) every day. The first thing I noticed was that my bowels moved more freely and I wasn't bloated anymore. Later I added kefir and kombucha to my routine for the probiotics. My gut never felt so good! I was really surprised to find how much better my skin looked too and how much better my clothes fit. I guess I'd just not given all that much thought to the idea of cleaning my "insides." My breast cancer changed all that.*

—Karla J., breast cancer survivor

# Chapter 10

# Hormone Harmony

*We are indebted to Dr. Jonathan Wright for his groundbreaking work on women's hormones and for allowing us to use his writings (wrightnewsletter.com) to express key concepts in this chapter.*

> CHAPTER GOAL: Balance your hormones

It seems as if every day, we hear more bad news about estrogen. Both medical journals and the popular press warn us about its dangers. In fact, after derogatory news about pharmaceutical hormone replacement emerged from the Women's Health Initiative in 2002, both the study and millions of women's prescriptions were abruptly halted (NIH 2002). Moving farther into the second decade of the century, the subject of hormone replacement remains a source of intense controversy.

As we dig deeper, we find a more nuanced story: it is not estrogen itself that is the problem; it's the type of estrogen to which we're exposed, how it is metabolized by the body, and how it dances with progesterone and other hormones that matters (Kabat et al. 2006). In this chapter we'll look closely at the facts, not the hyperbole, to help you sort through the evolving story surrounding this contentious hormone.

# Meet Your Estrogens

While many of us have traditionally thought of estrogen as a single hormone, it is actually a family of hormones comprising several distinct molecules that the body secretes naturally, the most well known of which are estrone (E1), estradiol (E2), and estriol (E3). Along with progesterone, testosterone, 5-dehydroepiandrosterone (or 5-DHEA, commonly known as DHEA), and corticosteroids, estrogens are in the steroid group of hormones that are all made from the same basic building block: cholesterol.

Of the three plentiful forms of estrogen just mentioned, estradiol is the most potent. Primarily a growth hormone, estradiol shapes tissue growth in the vagina, breasts, endometrium, fallopian tubes, ovaries, bones, and, of course, the developing fetus. Before menopause, most of your estradiol is produced by the ovaries, with lesser amounts produced by the adrenal glands, the liver, and the breasts. Fat cells also secrete estradiol; hence heavier women tend to carry it in greater concentrations.

Estrone, a weaker estrogen derived from estradiol in the liver, serves as a backup form of estrogen. Although we stop manufacturing most estradiol after menopause, the adrenal glands continue to produce estrone after menopause and for the rest of our lives.

The third key estrogen compound, estriol, plays *its* pivotal role during pregnancy, when levels of this "weak" estrogen start to soar. Although scientists have considered estriol to be too weak to be relevant except during pregnancy, it now appears that this "weakness" might actually be its strength.

One study (Siiteri et al. 2002) that suggested this was conducted in Berkeley, California, where researchers examined frozen blood samples of fifteen thousand women who had been pregnant forty years earlier. They found that of all the study subjects, those with the highest levels of estriol relative to other estrogens during pregnancy had the lowest occurrence of breast cancer. Specifically, women with the *highest* level of estriol during pregnancy had a 58 percent *lower* risk of developing breast cancer than the women with the *lowest* estriol levels. It's noteworthy that during pregnancy, estriol levels climb enormously, by one thousand times or more. Even after childbirth, estriol levels usually remain higher than they were before pregnancy.

To summarize, it's clear from the data that all estrogens are not the same. And it gets even more interesting than that.

## The "Daughter" Metabolites: E2, E4, E16

Over the last three decades, with evolving interest and tools, researchers have been paying fresh attention to an additional family of estrogen complexes. We might call them "daughter" metabolites because they are the estrogen by-products that emerge after estradiol, estrone, and estriol are processed, or detoxified, by the liver. The technical terms for these by-products are 2-hydroxyestrone (2-OHE), 4-hydroxyestrone (4-OHE), and 16$\alpha$-hydroxyestrone (16$\alpha$-OHE), and together they give us a very clear picture of whether the amounts and types of estrogen in your body are apt to cause trouble.

Once the body uses estrogen, like everything else, the estrogen heads to the liver for detoxification. Properly metabolizing and excreting estrogens, the essence of detoxification, is a critical but tricky task. If the estrogens are metabolized into 2-hydroxyestrone, they lose most of their aggressive activity; thus they are known as "good" estrogen metabolites. Research indicates that when levels of 2-hydroxyestrone are higher, the body resists cancer, and when these levels are low, cancer risk increases (Gaikwad et al. 2008). On the other hand, women who metabolize a larger proportion of their estrogens into 16α-hydroxyestrone and 4-hydroxyestrone show an elevated risk of breast cancer (ibid.).

Why would the liver use a pathway that could lead to adversity? Recall from chapter 9 that gut and liver health are intimately tied to estrogen metabolism. A liver that is compromised by toxicity, alcohol, or estrogen overload from environmental sources (see chapter 4), for example, will not do as good of a job at clearing out excess estrogen as a liver that's at the peak of health. Likewise, a healthy population of gut bacteria actually helps to detoxify excess estrogen (via the containment of an enzyme called *beta-glucuronidase*). In effect, these desirable microbes provide the "bug-power" to help carry excess estrogen out of the body.

Where's the proof? Examining this premise in context, among 10,786 premenopausal women studied in the 1990s, researchers observed that women who developed breast cancer had notably less 2-hydroxyestrone—a full 40 percent less—and more 16α-hydroxyestrone metabolites than women who did not develop breast cancer (Muti et al. 2000). Another study, this one on postmenopausal women, found that those with the highest ratio of estradiol to 16α-hydroxyestrone had a 30 percent lower risk of developing breast cancer than women with lower ratios (Meilahn et al. 1998). If we could only find a way to make sure the liver is turning out healthy estrogen metabolites, as opposed to unhealthy ones, we could lower our breast cancer risk. It turns out that we can, and we'll get back to that part of the estrogen story shortly.

## What Else Affects Our Estrogen Load?

To reiterate, it's not estrogen per se that is the problem for women. Estrogen has played a vital role in reproduction and female well-being since the beginning of humanity. But the amounts of estrogen that our bodies need to metabolize, as well as the types of estrogen that proliferate in excess, have steadily expanded in the chemically laden, hyper-estrogenic world of the twenty-first century.

As we discussed extensively in earlier chapters, animal estrogens from factory-farmed meat and dairy products, plus xenoestrogens from chemicals, plastics, pesticides, and other contaminants, can wreak havoc with our balance of *natural* estrogens. Estrogen also dances with other hormones, and the nature of the dance can influence breast-cancer risk in an equally dramatic way.

## ESTROGEN AND PROGESTERONE

Progesterone is a steroid hormone produced in the ovaries that is essential for normal breast development during puberty, for regulating the menstrual cycle, for maintaining a pregnancy, and for preparing for lactation and breastfeeding. While estrogen is the hormone that stimulates cell growth, progesterone is the hormone that inhibits growth, induces cell maturation, and initiates programmed cell death (apoptosis).

In his first book on natural progesterone, the late Dr. John Lee (2001) explains how "estrogen dominance" can affect women who have any amount of estrogen but have little or no progesterone to balance the effects of estrogen in the body. Please note that while synthetic progesterone (progestin), such as that used in the illustrious Women's Health Initiative study mentioned earlier, is considered to be carcinogenic, natural progesterone is thought to be protective; in fact, many researchers agree that healthy levels of progesterone in the body may actually help protect you against breast cancer (Jerry 2007).

But as we grow closer to menopause, our progesterone levels begin to wane, a decade or even more before estrogen wanes. Here is where the state of estrogen dominance becomes apparent: our bodies make too little progesterone in relationship to estrogen. Not surprisingly, this is when we become most susceptible to breast cancer. Also not surprisingly, this is when many women begin talking to their doctors about supplementing with natural progesterone.

## ESTROGEN AND THYROID HORMONE

The thyroid gland and estrogen share a close and somewhat complicated relationship. As on a seesaw, when one part is out of balance, it can readily throw the other one off as well. For instance, while an increase in estrogen does not lower production of thyroid hormones, it does cause a chain reaction that renders thyroid hormones less active. Fortunately, millions of women have been helped by research completed back in 1964, which established that adequate thyroid hormone helps estradiol metabolize more completely into the "good" estrogen metabolite, 2-hydroxyestrone (Fishman et al. 1965). Indeed, many, but not all, studies indicate that having an underactive thyroid slows the process of clearing estrogen from the body, thus creating a state of estrogen dominance, a known risk factor for breast cancer (Vasudevan, Ogawa, and Pfaff 2002). Clearly, this is an area that requires significantly more research and analysis. As always, we believe that balance is key: a thyroid gland that works properly—that is neither hyperactive nor hypoactive—will help keep the rest of your metabolism in balance. That is our goal!

## ESTROGEN AND MELATONIN

Sleep habits also influence estrogen levels. Melatonin, the "sleep hormone" that we produce when we sleep in complete darkness, helps reduce excessive estrogen production. By simply sleeping in a completely dark room (and avoiding working night shifts, if possible), you take another powerful step in keeping your estrogen levels under control.

## ESTROGEN, OBESITY, AND INSULIN

The current obesity epidemic has taken a toll on our hormonal balance, as reported in numerous journals over the past decade, including the *New England Journal of Medicine* (Yager and Davidson 2006) and the premier medical journal of the United Kingdom, the *Lancet* (Bianchini, Kaaks, and Vainio 2002). As we discussed in chapter 6, obese women have a higher risk of developing breast cancer for a variety of reasons. One key factor underlying this higher risk is an elevated level of circulating estrogens that is linked to greater amounts of adipose (fat) tissue. Adipose tissue serves as an additional site for estrogen production.

But there's another hormone at play here as well. The liver produces a hormone called *sex hormone–binding globulin* (SHBG), which carries sex hormones around the body and regulates their access to tissues. In women,

SHBG has a special affinity for estradiol; that is, the more SHBG we have, the more estradiol is "bound up." This is, by and large, a good thing.

Obese women have lower levels of SHBG, making more estrogen available to breast tissue. Perhaps most ominously, research published in the *Journal of Clinical Investigation* showed that a high-fructose diet (containing high-fructose corn syrup, for example, present in virtually all processed foods and beverages) decreased levels of SHBG in the liver by a whopping 80 percent, resulting in higher levels of circulating estrogen (Selva et al. 2007). Fortunately, a foundational Eating for Health plan, plus the specific suggestions in chapter 6, will go a long way toward helping manage excess weight and insulin, and, in the process, controlling levels of estrogen and SBGH. We'll provide several suggestions for lowering estrogen load later in this chapter.

# Assessing Your Status

Dr. Jonathan Wright, medical practitioner since 1973 and author or coauthor of twelve health books, including *Stay Young and Sexy with Bio-Identical Hormone Replacement* (Wright and Lenard 2010), was the first to introduce an integrated, balanced pattern of bioidentical hormones for women, in the early 1980s. He has been prescribing, researching, and writing about them ever since. In fact, much of what we know about the various forms of estrogen and their actions in the body is due to his exhaustive investigation on the issue. Here's what he has to say about assessing estrogen-related cancer risk.

First, Dr. Wright recommends a look at the "EQ" or *estrogen quotient*, a ratio first described by Dr. Henry Lemon of the University of Nebraska medical school. The EQ is the relationship of estriol to estradiol and estrone. The higher your EQ, mathematically derived as $E3/(E1+E2)$, the better. Dr. Lemon, the originator of the EQ test, and colleagues (1966) tested estriol along with estrone and estradiol by having women collect their urine for twenty-four hours and then measuring the hormone levels in the specimens.

With the authorization of a doctor, nutritionist, or other health professional, the testing kits can be mailed to you at home, where you collect your specimen and send it back to the lab. Remember, it's not the absolute amount of estriol that appears to be the most important number, but the relative amount of estriol compared with the sum of estradiol and estrone. According to Dr. Wright (2005), "In today's environment, with the amount of estrogen-mimicking carcinogens increasing dramatically, it's more important than ever to keep your level of estriol as high as possible. So I don't see any reason why we shouldn't…shoot for an EQ of 1.0 or above." Interestingly, Dr. Wright also discovered that iodine raises the EQ for nearly all women.

The second test Dr. Wright recommends is commonly called the "2:16," referring to the relationship of the estrogen metabolites we discussed earlier (2-hydroxyestrone and 16$\alpha$-hydroxyestrone). Testing the 2:16 ratio can be done separately or along with the EQ. You definitely want more "good" (2-hydroxyestrone) estrogen than "bad" (16$\alpha$-hydroxyestrone) estrogen—substantially more if possible; any ratio below 1.0 is unfavorable. Although there's no consensus concerning the ideal ratio, Dr. Wright recommends 2.0 or greater, if possible. This lab test will also report on your level of 4-hydroxyestrone, which also appears to have carcinogenic tendencies, as well as your level of another metabolite known as 2-methoxyestradiol, an extremely potent, natural anticarcinogenic form of estrogen made by all women's bodies. For information on where to obtain these lab tests, refer to appendix B.

## Breast Thermography: Visually Evaluating Estrogen's Effects on the Breasts

Blood and urine tests can provide information regarding estrogen that is circulating throughout the body, but the question remains as to how much actually ends up in the breast tissue. The amounts are certainly not the same; in fact, the concentration of estrogen in the breasts may be ten to fifty times the concentration in the bloodstream (Jefcoate et al. 2000).

Breast thermography offers a solution to this problem by providing an indirect way to visualize the effects of estrogen on the breasts. While it does not measure estrogen per se, a thermography exam can identify the type of blood vessel patterns that estrogen would commonly produce. Excessive levels of estrogen in the breast would normally produce a vascular pattern that is different from a breast with normal estrogen levels. If you are taking birth control pills or undergoing hormone-replacement therapy, a thermogram can be especially valuable to you to determine whether or not the estrogen you are taking is harming your breasts and increasing your cancer risk.

# Guidelines for Managing Your Estrogen Load

Because an overabundance of the wrong kinds of estrogens can place a burden of risk on your body, consider making it a top priority to lighten your estrogen load. Here are our suggestions for doing just that.

## Avoid Xenoestrogens

To beat this drum one last time, it is truly essential to be aware of estrogenic compounds (known also as xenoestrogens) in the environment, which are having a greater and greater impact on not only breast cancer rates but also all other cancer rates. In particular, avoid conventional meats and dairy products; pesticide-laden produce (see ewg.org/foodnews /summary/ for a list of the "dirty dozen" fruits and vegetables); plastic items, especially heated or frozen plastic containers and those made with BPA; and personal care products with ingredients you don't immediately recognize. In *Hormone Deception*, Lindsey Berkson (2000) discusses the effective use of low-heat saunas (which induce sweating) to help remove xenoestrogens. Also, curcumin—a powerful phytonutrient in the spice turmeric—is currently the subject of multiple studies, with preliminary research suggesting that it may also be effective for this purpose.

## Maintain a Healthy Estrogen-Progesterone Balance

Maintaining a healthy estrogen-progesterone balance is easier said than done. Many women have had wonderful results from using bioidentical progesterone creams or capsules, *not to be confused with progestins,* which are pharmaceutical progesterone-type drugs shown to *increase* breast cancer risk (Bluming and Tavris 2009). While the labels of many products on the market claim that they are progesterone creams, our view is that hormone balance is too critical to be left to chance. Therefore, we believe it's imperative that you work with an integrative practitioner to measure your progesterone levels so you can add just the right amount of bioidentical progesterone to maintain a healthy hormone balance.

Keep in mind that birth control pills only add to your body's estrogen load, making this balance even more difficult to attain.

## STRESS IS A PROGESTERONE BUSTER

Progesterone is the major precursor of important corticosteroid hormones (aldosterone and cortisol) made in the adrenal cortex. When progesterone is sidelined into producing cortisol, the hormone that helps us deal with physical and emotional stress, there's less progesterone available for other uses, such as balancing estrogen.

In this way, the fast-paced, demanding lifestyle of the twenty-first century can deprive the body of its natural progesterone, which already declines dramatically after menopause under any circumstances. Premenopausally, stress may also affect your ability to ovulate, restricting or shutting down the production of progesterone entirely.

## *Exercise Helps Reduce Estrogen Levels*

The results of over two dozen epidemiologic studies on exercise and estrogen levels show us that women who exercise regularly have a reduced risk of developing breast cancer (see, for example, Campbell and McTiernan 2007). Moreover, a 2002 study (Chlebowski, Aiello, and McTiernan) assessed the *direct* effect of exercise on estrogen levels and found that women who exercised and lost more than 2 percent of their initial body fat had a 14 percent decrease in estradiol levels. Is it the loss of body fat or the exercise itself that reduced estrogen levels in this study of postmenopausal women? The results don't tell us, but we do know that both a healthy weight and healthy estrogen levels are essential to managing breast-cancer risk. If exercise can accomplish one or both of these goals, we're in good shape!

# Think Before You Drink

Steering clear of excess alcohol intake is important, because the same liver enzymes that break down alcohol are also used to clear estrogen. What's more, excess alcohol consumption is linked to higher estrogen levels (Seitz and Maurer 2007).

# Reweighting Your Estrogen Ratios

An Eating for Health food plan, with its emphasis on fresh fruits and vegetables, will provide an excellent start for helping you to eliminate unhealthy estrogens (16α-hydroxyestrone and 4-hydroxyestrone) while raising levels of healthy estrogens (estriol and 2-hydroxyestrone). You'll want to pay particular attention to the foods and nutrients that follow.

## CRUCIFEROUS HEROES

Cruciferous vegetables, those belonging to the *Brassica* genus, are the quickest route to shifting your estrogen balance toward the favorable 2-hydroxyestrone estrogens. The power of this vegetable group has been demonstrated both in the lab (Pledgie-Tracy, Sobolewski, and Davidson 2007) and in population studies (Kim and Park 2009). Known for encouraging healthy liver detoxification and for shifting more estrone toward the "good" 2-hydroxyestrone pathway, this family includes broccoli and its sprouts, cauliflower, cabbage (red, white, and napa cabbage, as well as bok choy), Brussels sprouts, arugula, collards, kale, daikon radish, kohlrabi, rutabaga, turnip, and watercress.

Note that excessive consumption of raw vegetables in this group can cause thyroid trouble for some people; we suggest that you lightly steam these veggies and eat them raw only as an occasional treat.

## FIBER

Fiber is another key factor in the successful secretion of estrogens. In the absence of fiber to bind to, estrogen metabolites run the risk of being reabsorbed by the body. That's why eating a diet that is low in fiber, having a history of chronic constipation, or both are associated with excess estrogen. What's more, soluble fiber—found in fruits, vegetables, nuts, seeds, and legumes—is fermented in the colon to create healthful flora. Fiber also breaks down into a unique fatty acid known as *n-butyrate*, which is believed to have anticancer properties (McIntyre, Gibson, and Young 1993).

## LIGNANS

As you will recall from chapter 9, another reason to enjoy flaxseeds on a regular basis is that they contain high amounts of lignans, phytochemicals that, when acted on by healthful intestinal microbes, are transformed into the protective compounds enterolactone and enterodiol. These compounds may redirect estrogen metabolism toward a healthy ratio of 2-hydroxyestrone to 16$\alpha$-hydroxyestrone (McCann et al. 2004). Flaxseeds have also been shown to raise levels of SHBG (Hyman 2007), reducing the amount of free estrogen available to act on breast tissue.

Other good sources of lignans are sesame seeds, whole grains, and olives.

## FERMENTED FOODS

We've talked quite a bit about the brilliant contributions that beneficial organisms can make to your health and to your cancer defense team. But where do you find these profoundly benevolent bacteria? Fermented foods, overflowing with microflora, are a fabulous addition to your diet. If you're new to fermented foods, a good place to start would be organic yogurt. Keep in mind that the carb content of yogurt is normally lower than that of nonfermented dairy products, because the lactose (milk sugar) is digested by friendly bacteria as part of the fermentation process.

Perhaps you'd enjoy trying kombucha (fermented tea), amazake (fermented rice drink), or kefir (fermented milk). What about homemade sauerkraut (see the recipe in appendix B) or kimchi? They all contain copious amounts of cooperative microflora, which, as you know by now, we consider to be one of the keys to the kingdom of good health!

## FERMENTED SOY

Because fermented foods provide beneficial bacteria, we also recommend the consumption of moderate amounts of fermented, organic soy products, such as natto, miso, and tempeh. Although soy has a long and controversial history, its phytochemicals genistein and daidzein have been credited with helping to alter the 2:16 estrogen ratio, while the fermentation process helps to deactivate potentially troublesome goitrogens (substances that induce goiter formation). Soy falls into the category we call *phytoestrogens*, compounds that are estrogen-like, but actually compete with estrogen for territory on a cell's surface. This ability to bind to cell receptors *instead* of estrogen serves to prevent human estrogens and xenoestrogens (environmental estrogens) from attaching to cells and promoting growth (Tempfer et. al. 2007).

We do *not* believe that *processed* soy has this same positive effect. One study (Allred et. al. 2004), in fact, looked at the specific effect of soy processing and its impact on breast cancer. Animals with breast cancer were fed soy from various sources—from unprocessed soy foods to highly processed soy protein isolates—all containing the same amount of genistein. When all was said and done, the highly processed soy appeared to *promote* cancer growth. For this reason, we recommend against processed soy products, such as soy burgers, soy franks, soy ice cream, soy protein bars, and so on.

## EVE HAD IT RIGHT

Some scholars contend that it was a pomegranate, not an apple, that tempted Eve in the biblical Garden of Eden. While we'll never know for sure, we do know that eating pomegranates or drinking pomegranate juice may help prevent and slow the growth of ER+ breast cancer. A group of phytochemicals called *ellagitannins*, found plentifully in pomegranates, was shown to inhibit the growth of estrogen-responsive breast cancer in laboratory tests. The researchers (Adams et al. 2010) believe that it's the ellagitannins in pomegranates that work as natural *aromatase* inhibitors; aromatase is a key enzyme the body uses to make estrogen, particularly after menopause. Further studies will be needed to confirm this effect; meanwhile, we know that eating pomegranates and pomegranate products can help keep breast cancer at bay via several other possible mechanisms (see chapter 3).

## NUTRIENTS

High-quality, targeted supplements can also go a long way in helping you achieve the goal of maintaining a health-enhancing balance of estrogens in your body. The following are some of our favorites, although it is always best to work with a qualified nutrition professional or other holistic health care practitioner to create just the right balance for *you*.

**Calcium d-glucarate.** Calcium d-glucarate, a natural substance found in apples, oranges, broccoli, spinach, and Brussels sprouts, helps the liver with its job of detoxifying estrogens via a process known as glucuronidation. Calcium d-glucarate also helps inhibit the glucuronidase enzyme mentioned earlier, which in turn facilitates the elimination of estrogens. A typical dosage is 500 milligrams per day. Note that the mineral magnesium is the cofactor that helps this whole process run smoothly. Green, leafy vegetables; legumes; nuts; seeds; and whole grains are good sources of magnesium. Remember that when flour is refined and processed, the magnesium-rich germ and bran are removed.

**I3C or DIM.** Indole-3-carbinol, known by its close friends as I3C, is one of the key phytonutrients in cruciferous vegetables that gives them their estrogen-modulating effect. Eating broccoli sprouts, cauliflower, and other crucifers releases I3C, but you can also take it as a supplement for preventive therapy. Diindolylmethane, or DIM, a metabolite of I3C created when I3C mixes with juices in the stomach, is also used as a supplement for prevention. Both compounds are believed to work by promoting the formation of the healthful estrogen 2-hydroxyestrone.

**Methylation boosters.** *Methylation* is one of the biochemical pathways used by the liver to detoxify estrogens and other compounds, specifically raising 2-hydroxyestrone levels and lowering harmful 4-hydroxyestrone levels. For this reason and because there is a growing consensus that deficient methylation is a major contributor to not just cancer but also many major degenerative diseases, we want to do all we can to support healthy methylation. Cruciferous vegetables, the ultimate dietary multitaskers, help this process along, as do foods high in vitamins $B_6$, $B_{12}$, and folate. You'll get abundant amounts of these nutrients by Eating for Health and taking a high-quality foundational multinutrient.

Please note, however, that after age fifty, it becomes more difficult to absorb vitamin $B_{12}$ through the gut, and deficiency is common. Your doctor can check your $B_{12}$ status using simple blood tests. Some women can enhance $B_{12}$ levels through oral supplementation, while others need regular $B_{12}$ injections.

To get a rough idea of how well you are methylating, your doctor can check the *homocysteine* level in your blood, because elevated serum homocysteine is a classic sign of a methylation defect. Try the previous suggestions and retest. If your homocysteine remains stubbornly high (above 10 micromoles per liter), you'll want to consider adding other known methylation-enhancing nutrients like *trimethylglycine* (TMG), choline, or *S-adenosylmethionine* (SAMe).

**Vitamin D.** Vitamin D protects us from breast cancer in a variety of ways, and here's yet another. Aromatase, the enzyme that activates estrogen synthesis, is essential for the progression of ER+ breast cancer in postmenopausal women. This is why postmenopausal women are frequently prescribed aromatase-inhibiting drugs for estrogen-positive tumors.

Emerging evidence indicates that vitamin D "helps regulate the expression of aromatase in a tissue-selective manner" (Krishnan et al. 2010). In other words, it appears that vitamin D can limit the conversion of aromatase to estrogen in breast tissue but *not* in the bones, where it is needed to preserve bone density. Thus it would appear that vitamin D not only functions as a preventive but also has great potential as an adjuvant treatment to existing protocols. This is something to watch with excitement!

## To Do

Know your estrogens: find out the ratio of your "good" to "bad" estrogens. Take action to reduce undesirable estrogens:

- Maintain estrogen-progesterone balance
- Manage your weight and your glucose and insulin levels

- Avoid xenoestrogens wherever possible

- Eat lots of cruciferous vegetables, fiber, lignans, pomegranates, and fermented foods to help convert 16α-hydroxyestrone and 4-hydroxyestrone to 2-hydroxyestrone

- Keep levels of exercise *up* and levels of alcohol *down*

- Use targeted supplements such as calcium d-glucarate and IC3 as needed

- Support healthy methylation with B vitamins

- Manage aromatase conversion to estrogens with vitamin D

## Last Word

*I guess my "aha" moment came when I realized that what my doctor had been telling me for years about cholesterol was also true for estrogen: it could be both good and bad. This made immediate, intuitive sense to me, as I don't believe nature would have us carrying around hormones in our bodies that are there solely to make us sick. That knowledge was remarkably empowering, because I now have a way to see exactly how my hormones are contributing to my health picture, and know what changes I need to make if they become unbalanced.*

—Suzi G., breast cancer survivor

# AFTERWORD

A breast-cancer diagnosis is devastating for any woman, but after the treatment decisions are made and carried out, what happens next? I found myself in that position in May 1996. I chose mastectomies for my breast cancer after the excisional biopsy showed invasive ductal carcinoma in the form of a 1.5 centimeter tumor. The surgeon later said I had chosen the correct surgery because, at the time, he had not known that a second tumor of the same size was hiding deep in the breast. To help prevent recurrence, I chose an oophorectomy (ovary removal), but then what was I to do? This started my crusade to do whatever I could to prevent recurrence; and fear, faith, family, and friends, in various combinations, were with me every step of the way.

My cancer journey taught me to respect fear. That might sound a little strange, but fear became my friend because it was a great motivator. It helped me to reach the simple realization that everything I had done in my life up to that point had led to breast cancer, so everything had to change if I wanted to live.

I had started out as a "sugarholic," junk-food junkie, couch-potato worrywart. My intuition told me that my scare with cancer was a matter of life and death, so I made a lot of changes quickly. I found a wellness guide to advise me; underwent a cleanse; changed to a wellness diet and lifestyle; walked three miles, five times a week; and was put on a vitamin

regimen. For the first two years, Peter D'Adamo, a nationally known natu-
ropathic physician in Connecticut, guided my diet, as well as my supplement and herb intake. I also joined a wellness group and stayed with it for
fourteen years.

During that time, everyone in the group helped each other. Three of
us became long-term cancer survivors. We all shared with one another
what we had learned. To deal with my fear, I sought the help of a therapist,
underwent hypnosis, took a Silva meditation course, and listened to meditation tapes from Bernie Siegel to help with the sleepless nights.

About two years into my journey, I found *The Amazon Alternative
Therapies for Breast Cancer* LISTSERV (amazon-alternatives.org), an
online group of women with an approach to preventing recurrence similar
to the one I was taking. So these women from around the world became
my long-term friends, and we supported each other through our diet and
lifestyle changes. I learned early on to rely on the friends who supported
the many changes I continued to make as my journey progressed.

What allowed me to sustain my original momentum, which had
started with fear? A combination of knowledge, intuition, and faith in
myself and my higher power that I was on the right path. From the moment
of diagnosis, I read and studied everything I could get my hands on.
Understanding the physiology of the body and why I was doing what I was
doing made the changes enduring. When I understood how cancer feeds
on sugar, it became easy to replace sugar with fruit for my sweet tooth. The
funny thing about knowledge is that we can choose to ignore it, but we
can't take it away. No way was I going back to eating sugar and food additives and drinking impure water.

Also, when I realized that cancer didn't like oxygen, I could sense how
every step I took oxygenated my body, which made walking a pleasure.
I repeated a little mantra whenever I went walking. It changed daily but
went something like this: "I want to live, I want to be. I want to live, I want
to see." Learning to manage stress through meditation got me through
some very rough times.

Now you might be wondering how you can do it without some of the
resources I had. Throughout the years, I have seen many women recover
fully because they were committed to changing. It doesn't cost money to
walk, to learn to meditate, or to find friends, whether locally or online, to
help with support. Of course, eating a whole-food, organic diet can be

costly, but you can do this by finding local sources of organic food, growing your own, and being frugal with your decisions about what vitamin support you need.

I am reminded of a woman I knew through *The Amazon Alternative Therapies for Breast Cancer* LISTSERV. She was poor, with a diagnosis of stage 4 breast cancer and bones that looked like Swiss cheese. She studied hard on her own, bought over-the-counter nutritional supplements, changed her lifestyle, and lived for years and years.

At times I have been asked, "How do you stick to your wellness plan?" I still consider it a matter of life or death. But at the same time I have learned how to live in the real world. I do eat a sliver of birthday cake at family parties. And I eat a little bit of dark chocolate every day. I plan ahead by going to parties with a full stomach, and I've been known to take my own food. I also make wise choices when eating out. Most important, *my* choices have influenced my family and friends about their own choices, and this will affect their future health and that of their families.

I feel very blessed to have come this far, and realize that life is an ongoing journey. My children are married, and I am a grandmother of five. And my husband, who helped me to live, had me to help him through his final journey.

I can't say that the cancer walk is easy, but I know that if someone like me can change, then anyone can change.

—Marilyn Holasek Lloyd, sixteen-year breast-cancer survivor

# APPENDIX A

# HOW TO ENJOY EIGHT-PLUS SERVINGS OF VEGETABLES AND FRUITS EVERY DAY

*Used with permission, courtesy of Jeanne M. Wallace, PhD, CNC, Nutritional Solutions, Inc.*

Vegetables and fruits are excellent sources of vitamins, minerals, and fiber, which are essential for health. In addition, fruits and vegetables contain a class of nutrients called "phytonutrients" that are important for fighting cancer. Nearly four thousand phytonutrients have been discovered. To get the full spectrum of these cancer "phyters," you need to eat a wide variety of fruits and vegetables from every color of the rainbow.

A 2007 study (Moiseeva et al.) found that phytonutrients can "communicate" directly with our genes, altering genetic expression. They can suppress the response of cancer-causing genes known as *oncogenes* while *increasing* the expression of tumor-suppressor genes. Vitamin pills don't offer these important nutrients, so you'll want to substantially increase your intake of fruits and vegetables. Aim for eight to twelve servings per day. A serving is ½ cup of cooked vegetable; 1 cup of raw salad vegetables; 6 ounces of vegetable juice; 1 medium apple, pear, or other fruit; ½ cup diced, cooked, or canned fruit; or 1 cup of berries. Gradually increase your intake by one to two servings each week until you reach your goal. Here are some helpful tips:

- Plan to eat two or three ½-cup servings of vegetables at each meal (breakfast, lunch, and dinner). Snack on fresh fruits (or additional vegetables), and you'll surely meet your goal.

- Plan your meals around vegetables! Plant-based foods should fill 50 to 75 percent of your plate (with proteins and whole grains for the remainder).

- Be adventurous by expanding your horizons! Try a new fruit or vegetable each week. Have you tried kohlrabi, beet greens, star fruit, kiwi, celeriac, jicama, parsnip, fennel, bok choy, arugula, watercress, burdock root, fava beans, taro root, or mustard greens? Your grocery may provide recipe cards. It's easy to find recipes online if you're unsure of how to prepare your new find.

- Serve vegetable juices with meals and snacks for an easy way to boost your vegetable intake. Choose freshly made vegetable juice, preferably organic and low-sodium.

- Add ½ cup of finely shredded carrots to 1 cup of salsa. The crunchy texture adds a great spark to the salsa. Or try grated zucchini or summer squash.

- For breakfast, eat one or two eggs that are high in omega-3 (poached, boiled, or scrambled) with 1 cup of steamed green beans, spinach, arugula, kale, broccoli, zucchini, or other vegetables.

- Make an egg scramble for breakfast. Dice or shred any combination of onions, red or green peppers, and mushrooms. Sauté the vegetables in olive oil until they are tender. Add eggs. Season with turmeric (which results in a nice yellow color), garlic, thyme, oregano, nutritional yeast, pepper, other spices, or some combination of these ingredients.

- Make a breakfast burrito packed with pinto or black beans, onions, peppers, mushrooms, zucchini, and tomatoes.

- Try a fruit smoothie for breakfast. In a blender, purée ½ cup of green tea (or soy, rice, or almond milk; or organic low-fat yogurt or kefir), 1 tablespoon of whey protein powder, ½ banana, ½ cup of fresh berries, ¼ teaspoon of fresh lemon or orange zest, and 1 tablespoon of flaxseed meal. For variety, try mango-peach, tangerine-raspberry, pineapple-coconut, blueberry-nectarine, or any combination you desire!

- Incorporate more green, leafy vegetables into your diet. Choose spinach, Swiss chard, collards, kale, mustard greens, arugula, young dandelion leaves, or beet or turnip greens. Serve cooked greens with scrambled eggs or tofu for breakfast. Add a bunch of chopped greens to soups, stews, or salads. Mix chopped, cooked greens into hummus or other dips. (Fresh greens have more nutrition, but you can keep frozen spinach on hand for convenience.)

- Serve vegetable curries (broccoli, cauliflower, green beans, carrots, yams, and Brussels sprouts are great in curry).

- Serve fresh (or frozen) berries with plain low-fat yogurt for a snack or dessert.

- Grate the peel and pith from a fresh organic lemon or orange, and add the zest to oatmeal, muesli, cereal, whole-grain muffins, waffles, salads, or tea.

- Keep a bag of baby carrots, celery sticks, red pepper slices, and snap peas on hand for snacking. Serve with hummus, salsa, or bean dip.

- Expand the variety of vegetables in your salads beyond tomatoes and cucumber! Start with a variety of leafy greens. Banish iceberg lettuce, which is nutritionally "bankrupt," and choose romaine, red-leaf lettuce, mesclun, raw spinach, beet greens, and other dark, leafy greens. Top with ample chopped, diced, or grated vegetables. Add lots of different colors of vegetables for visual appeal! Try these vegetables in your next salad:

| | | | | | |
|---|---|---|---|---|---|
| avocados | cabbage, red or green | chickpeas | fennel | parsley | sugar snap peas |
| artichokes | | chives | garlic cloves, roasted | peas | |
| beets | carrots | daikon sprouts | | peppers, red or yellow | sunflower sprouts |
| broccoli | cauliflower | eggplant, grilled | green beans | radishes | watercress |
| broccoli sprouts | celery | | jicama | scallions | yams, grated raw |
| | chayote | fava beans | onion, red or white | | zucchini |

- For a treat, fresh fruit is nice for salads too. Try orange slices, raspberries, apple chunks, kiwis, pomegranate pearls, red grapes, mango, or grated orange or lemon zest.

- When baking muffins, cookies, or other treats, add grated carrots or zucchini to the recipe to boost fiber and carotenoid intake.

- Use applesauce or prune purée to replace half of the fat in baked goods. You can use puréed prunes (or baby-food prunes) to replace all the fat in chocolate brownies or baked goods. They add a chewy texture and a sweet flavor. Place ¾ cup of dried, chopped, pitted prunes in a blender and add 3 tablespoons of very hot water. Blend until the prunes are smooth.

- For a quick favorite family meal, top an organic frozen pizza with extra vegetables (onions, broccoli, red pepper, artichoke hearts, spinach, dried tomatoes).

- For a simple dinner, try roasted vegetables. Dice onion, leek, fennel, rutabaga, turnip, yam or sweet potato, zucchini, burdock root, red pepper, portobello mushrooms, peeled whole garlic cloves, and sprigs of fresh rosemary (optional). Toss with olive oil and roast uncovered in the oven at 375°F for 1 hour. Make extra; they are delicious as leftovers.

- Bake winter squash (acorn, butternut, or spaghetti squash). Make extra and store for a quick meal later in the week.

- Look for organic ready-made soups with simple ingredient lists in 1-quart boxes. Serve with salad for a quick lunch or snack. Or heat it in a cup and enjoy it as a warming beverage anytime.

- Add extra chopped vegetables and fresh minced parsley to ready-made tabbouleh.

- Make kebabs for the grill with zucchini, yellow squash, onions, mushrooms, cherry tomatoes, sweet peppers, eggplant, or pineapple wedges. (Grilling meats creates carcinogens called "HCAs" and is not recommended, but grilled vegetables are safe.)

- Combine 1 cup of cooked brown rice with 2 cups of diced vegetables (onions, carrots, zucchini, red peppers, mushrooms, or others). Season with garlic, thyme, and basil. Use this mixture to stuff bell peppers, cabbage rolls, and portobello mushrooms or squash halves. Bake until fragrant and tender.

- Prepare a big pot of homemade soup or stew (double the vegetables in the recipe) and a salad or vegetable casserole over the weekend. Later in the week, when you don't feel like cooking, a healthy meal is ready and waiting for you.

- If you eat organic meats, consider marinating them in fruit juices (try pomegranate, raspberry, or cranberry) or concentrated fruit purées (soak dried apricots or prunes in water to cover, and then purée in the blender). Add rosemary, garlic, ginger, black pepper, thyme, oregano, or other spices. Marinate overnight. Or try mixing ¼ cup of mashed blueberries or prune purée in each pound of ground bison (or organic, low-fat beef) for juicy burgers!

- When eating out, ask to have an extra serving or two of vegetables (without sauce) instead of bread, potatoes, or rice. And load up with lots of raw veggies at the salad bar, like dark-green lettuces (avoid iceberg) and spinach.

- Find yourself at a fast-food restaurant? Choose a salad and a baked potato topped with salsa.

- Add extra vegetables to soups, either homemade or canned.

- Make a quick "pasta salad" by adding 2 cups of cooked whole-grain rice, quinoa, amaranth, buckwheat, or other grain to 4 cups of diced vegetables and ½ cup of chopped fresh parsley. Make it as colorful as possible. Season with garlic, black pepper, and basil, and dress with olive oil and vinegar or lemon juice.

- For convenience, look to ready-to-eat (washed, peeled, sliced, grated, or some combination), packaged vegetables at the market. Or set aside some time on the weekend to wash and prepare vegetables for the upcoming week. Having containers of chopped onions, grated carrots, sliced zucchini, and other prepared vegetables on hand simplifies preparation of healthy meals.

- Put extra vegetables in spaghetti sauce. Try shredded carrots, onions, chopped spinach, roasted eggplant, mushrooms, or some combination of these ingredients.

- Make a stir-fry for dinner once a week. Cook a diverse assortment of vegetables over medium heat in 1/3 cup of broth and 1 tablespoon of olive oil (add a dash of sesame oil to jazz up the flavor).

- Bake an apple, quince, or pear for dessert. Core the fruit, stuff the center with a combination of uncooked rolled or steel-cut oats, cinnamon, chopped walnuts, and 1 tablespoon of raisins or currants. Bake at 375°F for about 45 minutes (the aroma will tell you when it's done).

# APPENDIX B

# YOUR EATING FOR HEALTH PANTRY AND RECIPES

## Setting Up an Eating for Health Pantry

(By Ed Bauman, PhD, and Lizette Marx, NC, from *Flavors of Health*, Bauman College Press, 2011)

### Dry Goods

Keep these foods in your cabinet or in a cool, dry place unless otherwise indicated. Some nuts and flours, for example, store best in the refrigerator or freezer. Ideal storage containers to use are mason jars or stainless-steel containers with tightly fitting lids. Spices are best kept in tinted-glass or stainless-steel containers.

# LEGUMES

| | |
|---|---|
| Adzuki beans | Black beans |
| Cannellini beans | Chickpeas |
| Fava beans | Kidney beans |
| Lentils | Lima (large and baby) |
| Mung beans | Pinto beans |

# WHOLE GRAINS

Whole grains do not keep as long as pearled or refined grains, because the germ portion of the kernels can cause the grain to become rancid over time. Never use grains or grain products that do not look or smell as they should. It is best to buy smaller quantities of grains and grain products to avoid discarding large amounts of grain due to spoilage.

| Grain | Storage Guidelines | Shelf Life |
|---|---|---|
| Amaranth | Store in a tightly sealed glass container in a cool, dark, dry location. Avoid cabinets near stoves, the oven, or the dishwasher. Avoid any warm location or sunlight, as grain will become bitter. | One year if stored properly |
| Barley | Store in a tightly sealed glass container in a cool, dark, dry location. Avoid cabinets near stoves, the oven, or the dishwasher. During the summer months, store in the refrigerator or freezer, making sure to seal the container or wrap the grain tightly to prevent moisture absorption from refrigeration. | One year if stored properly |

| | | |
|---|---|---|
| Basmati rice | Store in a tightly sealed glass container in a cool, dark, dry location. | Cabinet: two years if stored properly Refrigerator: indefinitely |
| Brown rice | Store in a tightly sealed glass container in a cool, dark, dry location, or in the freezer for longer periods. | Cabinet: one and one-half years if stored properly Freezer: two years or more |
| Buckwheat | Store in a tightly sealed glass or stainless-steel container in the refrigerator or freezer. Be sure to wrap the grain tightly to prevent moisture absorption from refrigeration. | Refrigerator: two to three months Freezer: six months |
| Corn | Store in a tightly sealed glass container in a cool, dark, dry location. | Several years |
| Millet | Store in a tightly sealed glass container in a cool, dark, dry location. For refrigerator or freezer storage, be sure the grain is tightly wrapped to prevent moisture absorption. If storing in a glass container with a tightly fitting lid, be sure container is filled completely. Partially filled containers pick up moisture from refrigeration. | Cabinet: two months Refrigerator: four months Freezer: six months or more |
| Oats | Store in a tightly sealed glass or stainless-steel container in a cool, dark, dry location. | One year if stored properly (the high levels of antioxidants in oats help to prevent spoilage) |

| Quinoa | Store in a tightly sealed glass or stainless-steel container in a cool, dark, dry location. | One year if stored properly; longer if stored away from sunlight and heat |
|---|---|---|
| Wild rice | Store in a tightly sealed glass container in a cool, dark, dry location. | Indefinitely if properly stored |

## PROCESSED GRAINS (FLOURS)

The refrigerator is a very good storage space for flour, but using a sealed container is even more important to prevent the flour from absorbing moisture as well as odors and flavors from other foods stored in the refrigerator.

The freezer compartment can be used for long-term storage, but when you are using a sealed container or a freezer bag, make sure it is full to eliminate as much air as possible.

Most types of flour can also be tightly wrapped for freezer storage, but wrapping is often an awkward method for storing large quantities. Wrap the flour tightly in plastic and then place it in a container with a tightly fitting lid, or wrap it again in aluminum foil.

Avoid refrigerating or freezing flour in its original paper packaging. Paper is porous, so the flour may absorb moisture and odors. But if the flour has not been opened, you can store the paper package in the refrigerator or freezer when it is tightly wrapped with plastic.

Properly stored flours will last from two to four months. Always allow flour to return to room temperature before using it for the best results. Flour that does not smell fresh should not be used.

| | |
|---|---|
| Brown rice flour | Buckwheat flour |
| Chickpea flour | Millet flour |
| Polenta | Quinoa flour |
| Spelt flour | Wheat flour |

## SEEDS

The best storage containers for nuts and seeds are those made of tinted glass or stainless steel. Flaxseeds in particular should be kept away from sunlight and heat. Ideally, flaxseeds should be refrigerated.

| | |
|---|---|
| Chia | Flax |
| Hemp | Pumpkin |
| Sesame | Sunflower |

## NUTS

Nuts contain a lot of oil and will go rancid easily if improperly stored. Store nuts in an airtight glass or stainless-steel container, and either refrigerate it or keep it in the freezer. Here are a few more guidelines for storing nuts:

- Let newly shelled nuts dry out for two to three days before putting them in the refrigerator or freezer to help prevent mold growth.

- Put nuts in a moisture-proof, airtight jar or wrap them tightly in a heavy plastic bag. This will help keep them from picking up odors from other foods.

- Store nuts in the refrigerator for up to four months. Sometimes they will stay fresh in the refrigerator for as long as a year.

- Store nuts in the freezer for up to nine months. Sometimes you can keep unsalted nuts in the freezer for as long as two years.

- Taste nuts before you use them to make sure that they are still good.

# RECIPES

## BANANA NUT QUINOA AND MILLET HOT CEREAL

(By Ed Bauman, PhD, and Lizette Marx, NC, from *Flavors of Health*, Bauman College Press, 2011)

Quinoa and millet are delicious when cooked low and slow in fresh almond-banana milk sweetened with dates and spiced with cinnamon. This warming, high-protein hot cereal will sustain you through a busy morning.

*Yields 4 servings*

**1 cup dry quinoa, rinsed and then soaked overnight in filtered water with 1 tablespoon lemon juice or whey**

1 cup dry millet, soaked overnight in filtered water with 1 tablespoon lemon juice or whey

4 cups nut milk (preferably almond, hazelnut, cashew, or coconut)

1 ripe banana, broken in two

2 dates, pitted and coarsely chopped

Pinch of sea salt

½ teaspoon ground cinnamon

2 tablespoons coconut oil or unsalted butter

1 tablespoon flaxseeds, ground or whole

1 tablespoon maple syrup (optional)

Drain the quinoa through a fine-mesh sieve and run filtered water through the grains for 2 minutes. Once the quinoa has been thoroughly rinsed, transfer it to a bowl and set it aside. Use a rubber spatula to scrape out any grains that may have stuck to the inside of the sieve.

Repeat this process with the millet, transfering it to a separate bowl until you are ready to use it.

In a blender, combine the nut milk with the banana and dates, and mix until smooth.

Transfer the mixture to a medium saucepan, add the sea salt, and bring it to a gentle boil over medium heat.

When the milk just begins to bubble, lower the heat slightly and add the millet. Cook on medium-low heat, stirring constantly, for about 10 minutes.

Add the quinoa and cinnamon, and cook the mixture until the grains are tender, about 8 to 10 minutes. If the cereal is too thick, thin it with a little filtered water.

Stir in the coconut oil or butter. Top the mixture with flaxseeds and drizzle it with maple syrup. Add more nut milk or some yogurt, if desired.

# HELAYNE'S DAD BOB'S BREGGSFAST SPECIAL

1 teaspoon fresh or dried parsley, oregano, thyme, and/or rosemary

2 eggs, soft boiled (cooled for 8 minutes in cold water)

1 slice gluten-free bread, or 10 to 12 gluten-free crackers, crumbled

1 tablespoon extra-virgin olive oil

1 to 2 tablespoons nutritional yeast

1 clove garlic, minced

Sea salt

Place all the herbs and crumbled crackers in a bowl.

Add the olive oil to the crumbled bread or cracker mixture.

Remove the eggs from their shells and place them in the bowl.

Sprinkle nutritional yeast, garlic, and salt to taste. Mix together lightly and enjoy.

# Vegan High-Protein Lentil and Millet Burgers with Cashew Sauce

(By Ed Bauman, PhD, from the *Bauman College Natural Chef Cookbook*)

Because lentils, millet, and sunflower seeds are some of the best sources of vegetarian protein, this is a high-protein vegan burger. The dairy-free sauce uses the booster foods miso and nutritional yeast.

*Yields 8 to 10 patties*

## Burgers

½ cup brown lentils

½ cup millet

1 ½ cups water

½ teaspoon salt

½ cup sunflower seeds, toasted and ground

½ cup minced cremini mushrooms

¼ cup minced red onion

3 cloves minced garlic

½ cup finely grated carrot

¼ cup chopped parsley

1 tablespoon tamari

2 tablespoons arrowroot powder

¼ teaspoon red pepper flakes (or more to taste)

1 teaspoon chopped thyme leaves

## Sauce

½ cup raw cashews, soaked overnight and drained

½ teaspoon onion powder

¼ teaspoon salt (or more to taste)

¼ teaspoon garlic powder

Pinch of white pepper

½ cup almond milk

1 tablespoon olive oil

2 tablespoons nutritional yeast

1 teaspoon miso

1 tablespoon lemon juice

# BURGERS:

Preheat the oven to 350°F.

Put the lentils in a pot and add enough water to cover them by 2 inches. Bring it to a boil and then reduce the heat to a simmer. Allow to simmer for about 40 minutes, until very tender, almost mushy.

After starting the lentils, put the millet in a pot with the measured water and salt. Bring this mixture to a boil, and then reduce heat to a simmer and cover. Allow it to simmer for 20 to 30 minutes, until the water is absorbed and the millet is soft, with a porridge consistency but not watery. If the millet is still watery, remove the lid and continue cooking until the water has evaporated.

Transfer the cooked millet into a large bowl and allow it to cool.

When the lentils have finished cooking, add them to the bowl with the millet and mash the two together with a potato masher until they are well combined.

Add the remaining burger ingredients and mix well. Taste and adjust the seasonings as necessary.

Form the mixture into ½-inch-thick patties and place them on a parchment-lined baking sheet. Put them in the oven and bake them for 20 minutes.

Remove the baking sheet from the oven and allow the burgers to cool completely for at least 20 minutes. As they do, make the sauce.

# SAUCE

Put the cashews in a blender and blend until finely ground.

Add the onion powder, salt, garlic powder, and pepper. Pulse a few more times to combine.

In a glass measuring cup, whisk together the almond milk and olive oil.

With the blender on low, gradually pour the milk mixture into the cashew mixture. Blend until smooth and creamy.

Blend in the nutritional yeast, miso, and lemon juice. Taste and adjust spices if necessary.

Just before serving, broil the burgers for about 3 minutes on each side, until they are golden brown and crispy. Watch closely to avoid burning them.

Serve the burgers immediately with the sauce.

# Spicy Winter Squash and Red Pepper Bisque

(By Lizette Marx, Bauman College Natural Chef Instructor and Nutrition Consultant)

> 4 red bell peppers
>
> 4 cup ghee or butter
>
> 1 garlic bulb
>
> 2 pound acorn, kabocha, or butternut squash
>
> 1 yellow onion, diced
>
> 1 teaspoon sea salt
>
> 2 teaspoons cumin seeds
>
> 1 teaspoon mustard seeds
>
> 1 4 teaspoons chili powder
>
> 1 teaspoon turmeric
>
> 4 teaspoon cinnamon
>
> 4 cup white wine
>
> 4 cups chicken stock or mineral broth
>
> 1 tablespoon butter
>
> 1 can 12–5 oz coconut milk
>
> 2 cup cilantro (optional)
>
> 4 cup pumpkin seed, toasted (optional)

Preheat the oven to 350°F. Line a baking sheet with parchment paper. Slice the red peppers in half and remove the white membrane and seeds. Place the peppers cut-side down on the baking sheet and brush them lightly with the melted ghee.

Cut 2 inch off the stem end of the garlic bulb and drizzle it with a teaspoon of melted ghee. Wrap the garlic in a square of foil, lined with parchment paper, and place it on the baking sheet next to the red peppers.

Carefully cut the winter squash in half and scoop out the seeds. Brush the cut side lightly with ghee and place it cut-side down on the baking sheet. Roast all vegetables for 1 hour.

Check the red peppers after 30 minutes; if the skins are bubbly and wrinkled, they are ready. Remove them from the oven, transfer them to a heat-proof glass bowl, and cover them with a lid or plate. Covering the peppers will make the skins easier to remove later.

While the squash continues roasting, heat the remaining ghee in a wide soup pot over medium to low heat. Add the onions, season lightly with sea salt, and cook gently until the onions turn golden. Add the cumin and mustard seeds, and cook the mixture for 5 minutes, until the seeds become very aromatic.

Stir in the chili powder, turmeric, and cinnamon, and continue cooking for another 1 to 2 minutes on low heat.

Deglaze the pan using the white wine, increase the heat to medium-high, and cook the mixture until most of the liquid has evaporated.

When the squash is easily pierced with a fork, remove it and the garlic from the oven. Allow them to cool for about 10 minutes or until they are easy to handle. Scoop out the squash and place it in a bowl. Squeeze out the garlic cloves into the same bowl. Remove the thin skins from the red peppers, chop them roughly, and place them in the same bowl. Add the entire contents of the bowl to the soup pot with the onions and spices.

Add the broth and cook over medium heat for 10 minutes.

Remove the pot from the heat. Using an immersion blender, purée the soup directly in the pot. If you're using a regular blender, fill it no more than two-thirds full and be sure to vent it so that the top doesn't pop off (either remove the pop-out center from the lid, or lift one edge of the lid and drape it with a clean towel).

Rinse the soup pot, return the blended soup to the pot, and add the butter and coconut milk. Stir the mixture together gently until the new ingredients are well incorporated. Taste and adjust the seasonings. Add sea salt and pepper to taste.

Serve as is or stir in chopped cilantro and top each serving with toasted pumpkin seeds.

# CURRIED CAULIFLOWER
# AND RED LENTILS

(By Mira Dessy, NE, from grainsandmore.blogspot.com, 2011)

Serve over brown rice or quinoa.

- 2 cups red lentils, rinsed
- 4 cups water
- 2 tablespoons grape seed oil
- ½ teaspoon yellow mustard seeds
- ½ teaspoon cumin seeds
- 1 large yellow onion, diced
- 2 cloves garlic, minced
- 1 teaspoon ginger, grated
- 1 tablespoon curry powder
- 1 teaspoon ground turmeric
- 2 cups organic tomato sauce
- ½ cauliflower, chopped into bite-size pieces
- 1 teaspoon sea salt
- 1 tablespoon minced fresh cilantro

Place the rinsed lentils in a stainless steel pot. Add the water and bring to a boil. Reduce the heat, cover, and simmer for 40 to 50 minutes.

Make the curry sauce while the lentils are cooking. If the lentils are done before the sauce is ready, take them off the heat and set them aside until it is time to add them to the sauce.

Using a large saucepan, heat the grape seed oil.

Add the mustard and cumin seeds to the hot oil. Cook for 1 minute, stirring constantly.

Add the onion and sauté until it is golden and slightly wilted.

Add the garlic, ginger, curry powder, and turmeric, and cook for 1 to 2 minutes.

Add the tomato sauce and cauliflower. Reduce heat to medium low, cover, and cook until cauliflower is al dente, approximately 7 to 9 minutes.

Add the cooked lentils, sea salt, and cilantro, and cook for 2 to 3 more minutes.

# RED CABBAGE SALAD

(By Sela Seleska, NC, from sausalitonutrition.com, 2011)

*Yields 4 servings*

**6 cups thinly sliced red cabbage**

**1 tablespoon minced garlic**

**1 tablespoon chicken or vegetable broth**

**½ cup chopped scallions**

**1 tablespoon peeled, minced fresh ginger**

**1 ½ tablespoons soy sauce**

**½ tablespoon rice vinegar**

**Salt**

**White pepper**

Let the sliced cabbage and minced garlic sit for 5 minutes to bring out their health-promoting properties.

Heat the broth in a large stainless-steel skillet. Add the cabbage, garlic, scallions, and ginger, and sauté over medium heat for 3 to 4 minutes, stirring frequently.

Add the soy sauce and rice vinegar. Season with salt and pepper to taste.

# Yam and Seed Spread

(By Ed Bauman, PhD, and Lizette Marx, NC, from *Flavors of Health*, Bauman College Press, 2011)

This spread replaces ham and cheese as a sandwich filling and can also be used as a dip.

*Yields 4 servings*

**3 yams**

¼ **cup sunflower seeds, ground**

¼ **cup sesame seeds, ground**

¼ **cup poppy seeds, ground**

¼ **cup flaxseeds, ground**

¼ **cup yogurt**

½ **teaspoon cinnamon**

½ **teaspoon coriander**

½ **teaspoon peeled, ground fresh ginger**

½ **teaspoon sea salt**

Bake the yams at 450°F for 45 to 60 minutes or until soft.

Remove the skins and mash the yams.

Add the ground seeds.

Fold in the yogurt, cinnamon, coriander, ginger, and salt.

# HERBED SALMON

(Bauman College Natural Chef Program recipe)

What makes this recipe so good is that the natural fat in the salmon isn't cooked away by high heat, so the fish stays very moist. The skin helps promote this process by sealing in juices, and also contributes a flavor of its own. More or less fish can be used. Just adjust the other ingredients accordingly.

**Dash of extra-virgin olive oil**

**6 (5-ounce-thick) salmon fillets with skin**

**Pinch of salt**

**Pinch of pepper, freshly ground**

**2 tablespoons finely grated lemon zest**

Preheat the oven to 350°F. Gently rub a little olive oil into the flesh side of the salmon and season it lightly with salt and pepper. (Rubbing the fish will also give you the chance to feel for any small bones, which you can pick out with your fingers or a pair of tweezers.)

Lay the salmon skin-side down on a nonstick, oiled, or parchment-paper-lined baking sheet. Combine the herbs and the zest, and sprinkle them over the top of the fish, gently pressing into the flesh.

Reduce the oven temperature to 325° and roast the fish for 20 to 25 minutes, until it is just cooked through but still slightly translucent in the very center (check it with the tip of a knife). Serve the fish warm or at room temperature.

# Vegetable Biryani

(By Ed Bauman, PhD, and Lizette Marx, NC, from *Flavors of Health*, Bauman College Press, 2011)

   1 tablespoon and 2 tablespoons ghee or coconut oil

   2 cups brown basmati rice

   Pinch of saffron

   ¼ teaspoon turmeric powder

   ½ teaspoon salt

   4 cups vegetable stock

   1 ½ cups chopped yellow onion

   1 large carrot, diced

   1 cup chopped cauliflower

   1 tablespoon peeled, grated fresh ginger

   2 teaspoons ground cumin

   2 teaspoons ground coriander

   ½ teaspoon ground cinnamon

   Pinch of cayenne pepper

   ¼ cup water

   1 cup canned or fresh tomatoes, chopped, blanched, and peeled

   1 cup fresh or frozen peas

   1 cup chopped fresh greens (such as kale or chard)

   ⅓ cup cashews or Brazil nuts, toasted, for garnish

   ½ cup cilantro leaves, for garnish

Heat 1 tablespoon of the ghee in an 8 to 12-inch stainless steel or cast iron skillet and add the rice. Sauté briefly, stirring to coat each grain.

Add the saffron, turmeric, salt, and vegetable stock. Bring the mixture to a boil, cover, and reduce heat.

Simmer the rice mixture for about 50 minutes, until the liquid is absorbed and the rice is tender.

While the rice is cooking, heat the remaining 2 tablespoons of ghee in a separate 8-inch stainless steel or cast iron skillet over medium-high heat. Sauté the onions for 5 minutes, until tender.

Add the carrots, cauliflower, ginger, cumin, coriander, cinnamon, and cayenne pepper, and cook for 1 minute, stirring constantly.

Add the water and cover. Reduce the heat and cook for 3 to 4 minutes.

Add the tomato, peas, and greens. Simmer the mixture until the carrots are just tender.

Transfer the cooked rice to a bowl and fluff with a fork.

Add the onion and spice mixture to the rice, and mix well.

Transfer to a serving platter. Garnish with the nuts and cilantro.

# IMMUNE RECOVERY SOUP

Bauman, PhD, and Lizette Marx, NC, from *Flavors of Health*, Bauman College Press, 2011)

This is Mom's chicken soup, only more nutritious. If you're recovering from an illness, an infection, or exhaustion, drink 1 or 2 cups of immune recovery broth per day. You can also freeze single servings in small freezer bags and reheat them when you need a pick-me-up.

*Yields 8 servings*

## CHICKEN BROTH

1 cup dried organic lentils

½ chicken with bones

1 cup diced winter squash

1 tablespoon peeled, grated fresh ginger

1 tablespoon grated fresh turmeric

1 tablespoon grated fresh daikon radish

8 cups vegetable stock

## VEGETABLE FLAVORS

2 tablespoons olive oil

1 bulb garlic, peeled and chopped

2 onions, finely diced

2 red bell peppers, finely diced

6 shiitake mushrooms, sliced

1 cup shredded kale

1 bunch fresh parsley, chopped

1 bunch fresh cilantro, chopped

1 bunch fresh dill, chopped

1 bunch fresh thyme, chopped

# MINERAL AND SPICE SEASONING

**2 teaspoons seaweed (arame, hijiki, or dulse)**

**2 tablespoons curry powder**

**½ cup miso**

Place all the ingredients for the chicken broth in a large pot. Bring the broth to a boil, reduce the heat, and allow it to simmer for 2 hours.

Remove the chicken and let it cool.

Pick off the meat in shreds and set it aside.

Heat a large skillet over medium heat. Add the olive oil, garlic, onions, bell peppers, mushrooms, and kale. Sauté until the vegetables are tender, about 5 minutes.

Turn down the heat on the soup pot, being careful to avoid boiling the soup. Add the sautéed vegetables, reserved chicken, parsley, cilantro, dill, thyme, seaweed, curry powder, and miso.

# VEGETABLE PAD THAI

(By Ed Bauman, PhD, and Lizette Marx, NC, from *Flavors of Health*, Bauman College Press, 2011)

Thailand's national dish, pad Thai is often served as street food. Gluten-free, flat rice noodles are stir-fried with bean sprouts and a mixture of pungent fish sauce and sour tamarind. You must work fast, so make sure to prepare and lay out all of your ingredients before beginning to cook.

*Yields 6 servings*

1 (8-ounce) package pad Thai rice noodles

½ cup boiling, filtered water

2 tablespoons tamarind paste or soaked and puréed dried apricots

¼ cup palm, date, or organic cane sugar

¼ cup fish sauce (organic) or tamari

¼ cup filtered water

¼ cup brown rice vinegar

1 teaspoon chili powder

2 eggs, beaten

Pinch of salt

2 tablespoons coconut oil, ghee, or peanut oil

2 large shallots, minced

4 cloves garlic, minced

2 cups fresh bean sprouts

3 scallions, finely chopped

1 cup shredded daikon radish

¼ cup finely chopped peanuts or almonds

1 cup chopped cilantro

1 fresh lime, sliced

Cover the dry noodles with the boiling water and set aside for about 1 hour while you prepare the rest of the dish. When the noodles are softened, drain them and set them aside.

Place the tamarind paste or apricot purée in a saucepan over medium heat. Add the palm sugar, fish sauce, water, vinegar, and chili powder. Simmer this mixture until the palm sugar dissolves. Turn off the heat and set the pan aside.

Whisk the eggs and salt in a bowl.

Heat a skillet over medium-to-high heat and add 1 teaspoon of coconut oil. After the oil has melted, pour in the eggs. Allow them to set and then scramble them, breaking them into small pieces. Transfer the eggs to a plate and set it aside.

Have all of the remaining ingredients prepared and organized next to the stove.

Heat a wok or pan over medium heat and add the remaining coconut oil. Immediately add the shallots and garlic, and stir them until they start to brown, about 3 minutes, ensuring that they don't burn.

Add the noodles to the wok. Stir and toss them quickly to keep them from sticking.

Add the tamarind sauce and stir the mixture, being careful to avoid over-mixing the noodles, which would result in clumping. Cook the mixture until the liquid evaporates, about 5 minutes.

Toss the scrambled egg pieces into the pad Thai noodles.

Add the bean sprouts, scallions, and radish, and gently stir the mixture a few more times. The noodles should be soft but not mushy.

Transfer the mixture onto a serving plate and sprinkle it with the nuts and cilantro. Garnish it with a sliced lime and eat it while it is warm.

# HELAYNE'S FLOURLESS DARK CHOCOLATE TORTE

*Yields approximately 8 servings*

1 cup black beans, soaked overnight and cooked, or one 15-ounce can black beans, drained and rinsed

1 bar chocolate (eight 1-ounce squares dark chocolate, at least 70 percent cacao)

2 teaspoons pure vanilla extract

⅔ cup Grade B maple syrup

1 cup extra-virgin coconut oil

3 eggs

Preheat the oven to 350°F. Butter an 8-inch round cake pan and set it aside.

Place the beans in a food processor or blender and mix until smooth.

Using a double boiler or a small saucepan over very low heat, melt the chocolate with the vanilla extract.

In a large bowl, cream the maple syrup and coconut oil together until they are well combined.

Beat in the eggs, one at a time.

Combine the beans, chocolate, and coconut oil and mix well. Pour the mixture into the buttered cake pan and bake for 50 to 60 minutes or until the torte moves slightly when the pan is shaken.

Cool for 10 to 15 minutes before cutting and serving.

# HELAYNE'S ANTIOXIDANT SMOOTHIE

2 tablespoons green powder (such as NanoGreens)

12 ounces green tea, almond milk, or coconut water

½ cup berries

1 tablespoon pomegranate concentrate

1 banana

1 teaspoon maca powder

1 tablespoon nutritional yeast

½ to ¾ cup whole milk yogurt with active cultures

½ ripe avocado

1 teaspoon cod liver oil

1 scoop whey, rice, or hemp protein powder (optional)

Place all ingredients in a blender or food processor, and blend until smooth.

# LAURA'S ANTI-INFLAMMATORY LEMONADE

By Laura Halpin, N. C.

**1 cup lemon juice (4 to 6 lemons), freshly squeezed**

**4 to 6 cups filtered water (as desired)**

**1 teaspoon ground turmeric**

**1 teaspoon cinnamon**

**Pinch of healthy salt with iodine (such as Himalayan salt)**

**5 leaves fresh mint, julienned (optional)**

**½ teaspoon stevia (to taste)**

**½-inch slice fresh ginger, grated (optional)**

Stir all ingredients together until well mixed. Serve plain or over ice.

# LIVER TONIC TEA

(By Ed Bauman, PhD, and Lizette Marx, NC, from *Flavors of Health*, Bauman College Press, 2011)

Enjoy this tea infusion hot, at room temperature, or cooled over ice.

**¼ cup peeled, grated fresh turmeric root or 1 tablespoon ground turmeric**

**2 tablespoons peeled, grated fresh ginger root**

**1 teaspoon dried licorice root**

**2 teaspoons dried nettles or 2 nettle-leaf tea bags**

**4 cups water, cool and filtered**

**1 lemon**

**1 teaspoon raw honey (optional)**

Place turmeric, ginger, and licorice roots into a medium pot. Cover with the water. Bring the mixture to a boil and simmer it for 15 to 20 minutes.

Add the nettles and allow to steep for 10 minutes.

Strain the mixture into a clean, heat-proof glass container. Allow the mixture to cool for about 5 minutes.

Juice the lemon and pour into the tea along with a little honey, if desired.

# CHINESE IMMUNE TONIC TEA

(By Ed Bauman, PhD, and Lizette Marx, NC, from *Flavors of Health*, Bauman College Press, 2011)

This infusion of Chinese herbs provides powerful immune support. If these herbs are unavailable locally, you can order them online from reputable companies such as Starwest Botanicals (www.starwest-botanicals .com) or Mountain Rose Herbs (mountainroseherbs.com).

¼ **cup reishi mushrooms, sliced**

¼ **cup jujube dates**

¼ **cup rehmania root**

¼ **cup codonopsis**

¼ **cup astragalus root**

1 **teaspoon licorice root**

2 **quarts water, filtered**

Place all the herbs in a 4-quart pot and cover with the water. Bring the mixture to a boil and then reduce the heat to a simmer. Cook for 1 hour.

Strain the tea through a fine mesh strainer and serve hot, or cool to room temperature.

# GOOD-TO-THE-BONE BROTH

(By Ed Bauman, PhD, and Lizette Marx, NC, from *Flavors of Health*, Bauman College Press. 2011)

Featured in many traditional diets throughout the world, bone broths are highly nourishing and can add nutrients to a variety of dishes.

- 2 pounds bones from organic chicken or grass-fed beef, rinsed with filtered water
- 2 tablespoons apple cider vinegar or lemon juice
- 2 stalks celery, diced
- 2 large carrots, scrubbed and diced
- 1 large onion, diced
- 1 large leek, white part only, sliced
- 3 garlic cloves
- 5 peppercorns

# Bouquet Garni

**3 sprigs fresh thyme**

**1 leek stem (green portion of leek, about 5 inches long), cleaned**

**½ bunch parsley**

**1 bay leaf**

Preheat the oven to 400°F. Place the bones on an oiled or parchment paper–lined baking sheet and roast them until browned, about 30 minutes.

With a string, tie together the thyme, leek stem, parsley, and bay leaf to create the bouquet garni.

Add the roasted bones to a stockpot with the vinegar or lemon juice and just enough filtered water to cover the bones completely. Let stand for 30 minutes.

Bring stock to just under a boil and reduce heat immediately to simmer gently. Add the bouquet garni to the stockpot. Skim off any scum that rises to the surface. Add the celery, carrots, onion, leek, garlic, and peppercorns to the bone broth with an additional quart of water. Allow to continue simmering for at least 6 hours and as long as 48 hours (the longer this broth simmers, the better). Add more water as needed.

When the stock is finished, strain it through a fine mesh strainer lined with cheesecloth into a large bowl. Press the solids to extract as much liquid as possible.

Place the bowl of hot stock on ice to cool. Store the cooled stock in mason jars or use it in a recipe. Store in refrigerator for one week or freeze for up to 6 months.

If you freeze the stock, be sure to leave 2 inches of space from the top of the mason jar.

# Basic Sauerkraut

(By Sandy Der, taodekitchen.com)

**2 ½ pounds cabbage**

**1 ounce sea salt**

Make sure all equipment (bowls, spoons, knife, cutting board, jars, and so on) are clean. Remove all rings from your fingers and wash your hands well.

Shred the cabbage using a mandolin, or thinly slice it with a knife.

Place the cabbage in a large bowl. Toss the cabbage with the sea salt and mix well.

Using your hands, "knead" the cabbage until the natural juices are released and the volume of cabbage decreases. Alternatively, you can pound the cabbage with a blunt object to achieve the same effect. This will take 5 to 8 minutes.

Using a wooden spoon or potato masher, pack the cabbage into a crock or large jar (you can also divide the batch into a few smaller jars).

Weight down the cabbage with Pickle Weights, a small plate, or a clean rock.

Make sure there is enough cabbage brine to cover the cabbage. If you need more brine, dissolve 2 teaspoons of sea salt in 2 cups of water and add it to the crock.

Cover the mixture loosely with plastic and set it in a cool, dark place to ferment. Avoid storing the fermenting cabbage at temperatures below 55°F or over 76°F, or fermentation may not take place and the cabbage may spoil. Fermentation will happen more quickly in a warm environment.

After a week or two, start to taste the saeurkraut, and refrigerate it as soon as it is as sour as you like.

# Sweet Spice of Life

(By Ed Bauman, PhD, and Lizette Marx, NC, from *Flavors of Health*, Bauman College Press, 2011)

A classic Eating for Health spice that adds aroma and zest to your food, this is great sprinkled on smoothies, fruit, yogurt, and desserts.

> **4 tablespoons cinnamon**
>
> **1 tablespoon cardamom**
>
> **3 tablespoons ginger powder**
>
> **2 teaspoons nutmeg**
>
> **2 teaspoons allspice**
>
> **2 tablespoons dried orange peel**

Mix all of the spice powders and orange peel together. Store the mixture in an airtight container.

# RESOURCES

## Books

Barnard, N. D., and J. K. Reilly. 2008. *The Cancer Survivor's Guide: Foods That Help You Fight Back.* Summertown, TN: Healthy Living Publications.

Blaylock, R. L. 2003. *Natural Strategies for Cancer Patients.* New York: Kensington Publishing.

Block, K. I. 2009. *Life Over Cancer: The Block Center Program for Integrative Cancer Treatment.* New York: Bantam Books.

Brownstein, D. 2008. *Iodine: Why You Need It, Why You Can't Live without It.* 3rd ed. West Bloomfield, MI: Medical Alternatives Press.

Emeka, M. L. 2008. *Cancer's Best Medicine: A Self-Help and Wellness Guide.* 2nd ed. Port Orchard, WA: Apollo Publishing International.

Katz, R. 2008. *One Bite at a Time: Nourishing Recipes for Cancer Survivors and Their Friends.* With M. Edelson. Berkeley, CA: Celestial Arts.

———. 2009. *The Cancer-Fighting Kitchen: Nourishing, Big-Flavor Recipes for Cancer Treatment and Recovery.* With M. Edelson. New York: Ten Speed Press.

Moss, R. W. 1995. *Questioning Chemotherapy.* New York: Equinox Press.

———. 2000. *Antioxidants against Cancer.* New York: Equinox Press.

Murray, M. 2002. *How to Prevent and Treat Cancer with Natural Medicine.* New York: Riverhead Books.

Nixon, D. W. 1996. *The Cancer Recovery Eating Plan: The Right Foods to Help Fuel Your Recovery.* New York: Three Rivers Press.

Pendergrast, R. 2010. *Breast Cancer: Reduce Your Risk with Foods You Love.* North Augusta, SC: Penstokes Press.

Quillan, P. 2005. *Beating Cancer with Nutrition.* 4th ed. With N. Quillan. Includes CD-ROM. Carlsbad, CA: Nutrition Times Press.

Servan-Schreiber, D. 2009. *Anticancer: A New Way of Life.* New York: Viking Penguin.

Silberstein, S. 2005. *Hungry for Health.* West Conshohocken, PA: Infinity Publishing.

———. 2009. *Breast Cancer: Is It What You're Eating or What's Eating You?* Wynnewood, PA: Center for Advancement in Cancer Education.

Somers, S. 2009. *Knockout: Interviews with Doctors Who Are Curing Cancer.* New York: Three Rivers Press.

Thomson, P. A. J. 2006. *After Shock: From Cancer Diagnosis to Healing.* New Paltz, NY: Roots and Wings.

Weil, A. 2004. *Natural Health, Natural Medicine: The Complete Guide to Wellness and Self-Care for Optimum Health.* New York: Houghton Mifflin Company.

Yance Jr., D. R. 1999. *Herbal Medicine, Healing, and Cancer: A Comprehensive Program for Prevention and Treatment.* With A. Valentine. Chicago: Keats Publishing.

# Websites

## Advanced BC
**advancedbc.org**

Informational website about metastatic breast cancer support, advocacy, and resources

*American Association for Cancer Research*
**www.aacr.org**
Listings of cancer treatment, support, and research agencies

*American Cancer Society: Stay Healthy—Guide to Quitting Smoking*
**www.cancer.org/Healthy/StayAwayfromTobacco/**
**GuidetoQuittingSmoking/index**
Information to help quit smoking

*Annie Appleseed Project*
**annieappleseedproject.org**
Information, education, advocacy, and awareness about complementary
and alternative medicine for people with cancer

*Army of Women*
**www.armyofwomen.org**
A partnership between the Dr. Susan Love Research Foundation and
Avon Foundation for Women, working toward finding a cure

*Beat Breast Cancer through Breast Health*
**drsherri.wordpress.com**
Dr. Sherry Tenpenny's blog, sharing information, links, and scientific
reports

*Breast Cancer Choices*
**breastcancerchoices.org**
Information for patients to make informed choices about breast
procedures and treatments

*Breast Cancer Fund*
**breastcancerfund.org**
Breast cancer information site that highlights environmental causes of
breast cancer to help eradicate them

*Breast Equity*
**strittermed.org/breast_equity/**
Information about cancer news and research from Dr. Gwen Stritter

## Campaign for Safe Cosmetics, The
**safecosmetics.org**

Coalition that provides information about ingredients in cosmetics

## Cancer Avenues
**www.canceravenues.com**

Support and advocacy to help people who are seeking information about treatments, supplements, and research into breast cancer

## Cancer Decisions
**cancerdecisions.com**

Website of Ralph Moss, offering news, opinion, and treatment options regarding various topics related to cancer

## CanHelp
**canhelp.com**

Alternative cancer therapy organization helping to find therapy, counseling, and support for people who are seeking nonconventional treatment

## Center for Advancement in Cancer Education
**www.beatcancer.org**

An educational center providing information, counseling, and referral services for cancer prevention and support during treatment

## Centers for Disease Control and Prevention
**cdc.gov**

Links to various environmental health sites

## Cristiana Paul
**cristianapaul.com**

Guide to anti-aging, nutrition, and wellness information

## Dr. Susan Love Research Foundation
**dslrf.org/breastcancer/**

Information about prevention, detection, treatment, and surviving cancer

*EarthRose Institute*
**http://earthrose.org**

An informational organization working to help prevent exposure to toxins and provide information and education

*Environment, Health, and Safety Online*
**ehso.com**

Information about women's health and environmental links

*GrassrootsHealth*
**grassrootshealth.net**

Information and research about vitamin D

*Green Facts*
**www.greenfacts.org**

Information on endocrine disruptors and scientific reports that is accessible and understandable to the layperson

*Healing Cancer Naturally*
**healingcancernaturally.com**

A holistic view of cancer treatments with references to books, websites, and alternative therapies

*Iodine Group, The*
**iodine4health.com**

Website providing information on iodine and its effect on the body

*National Cancer Research Foundation*
**ncrf.org**

Information about cancer approaches that differ from conventional methods

*1 Up on Cancer*
**www.1uponcancer.com**

An online source of information on cancer, treatments, and resources aimed at survivors and bloggers

*Organic Consumers Association*
**organicconsumers.org**
Organization that supports organic food, food safety, labeling, farming, and sustainability

*Silent Spring Institute*
**silentspring.org**
Research on environmental links to breast cancer, environmental health, and the new field of green chemistry

*Silent Spring Institute: Environment and Breast Cancer—Science Review*
**sciencereview.silentspring.org/mamm_browse.cfm**
An online database reviewing mammary carcinogens

*Society for Integrative Oncology*
**www.integrativeonc.org**
Organization that promotes the scientific study of integrative treatment options, complementary therapies, and botanicals for cancer patients

*Sunlight, Nutrition, and Health Research Center*
**sunarc.org**
Organization that promotes changes in diet and lifestyle to help prevent chronic disease

*Think Before You Pink*
**thinkbeforeyoupink.org**
A project of Breast Cancer Action promoting accountability and responsibility in breast-cancer fund-raising

*Toxic Effects: Everyday Exposures*
**www.everydayexposures.com**
Information about toxins in and around the home and strategies for limiting your exposure

*Wellness Directory of Minnesota: Breast Cancer*
**www.mnwelldir.org/docs/cancer2/breast.htm**
Online wellness directory with information on attacking and preventing cancer, and boosting the immune system

*Weston A. Price Foundation, The*
**www.westonaprice.org**
Foundation promoting education and research toward restoring nutrient-dense foods to the diet

# Tests Referred to in This Book

| Type of Test | Purpose |
|---|---|
| 25(OH)D | 25-hydroxyvitamin D test measures through blood draw how much vitamin D is in your body. |
| C-reactive protein (high sensitivity) (HS-CRP) | CRP increases in the presence of inflammation. This test examines the levels of CRP through blood draw. |
| Fibrinogen | An important contributor to blood clotting, fibrinogen levels increase in response to tissue inflammation. Tests through blood draw. |
| HA1c | Measures blood sugar levels (hemooglobin A1c) over the last two to three months. Tests through blood draw. |
| Fasting insulin (FI) | Blood test that measures fasting insulin and helps assess insulin resistance or elevated cancer risk due to high insulin. |
| Ferritin | Ferritin is a protein produced in the liver for the storage of iron. Too much ferritin has an oxidizing effect on tissues and, therefore, the ferritin level should stay in the low to normal range for cancer survivors. Test is conducted through blood draw. |
| Total iron binding compound (TIBC) | Used to evaluate the ability of the protein transferrin to carry iron in the blood. |

| | |
|---|---|
| Ceruloplasmin and serum copper | Ceruloplasmin is a protein produced by the liver that binds copper for transport in the blood. Blood testing for ceruloplasmin with serum copper gives an indication of whether copper levels are in an appropriately low range for cancer survivors, since copper facilitates angiogenesis. |
| **Type of Test** | **Purpose** |
| Homocysteine | Measures levels of the amino acid homocysteine, which, in high amounts, can indicate defective methylation, a cellular process vital for detoxification. Conducted through blood draw. |
| Nutrient sufficiency | Combination of blood and urine tests that can assess status of B vitamins; CoQ10; vitamins C, E, and K; calcium; selenium; and many other nutrients. Offered by SpectraCell Laboratories and others. |
| Fatty-acid testing | Shows varying patterns identifying essential fatty-acid deficiency or excess, pro-inflammatory factors, or omega-3 dominance. Offered by Metametrix Clinical Laboratory and others. |
| Toxicity testing | Various panels examine exposure to environmental pollutants, including pesticides, PCBs, solvents, phthalates, heavy metals, and more. Offered by Metametrix Clinical Laboratory and others. |
| Comprehensive metabolic profile (CMP) | A combination urine, blood, and saliva test that assesses liver and neurotransmitter function, as well as cellular energy. Offered by Designs for Health and others. |
| Gastrointestinal (GI) function | Examines whether pathogenic (bacteria, virus, parasite) activity is present in the gut, the presence or absence of healthy gut flora, adequate digestive enzyme production, intestinal inflammation, and more. Offered by Diagnos-Techs and others. |

| Food allergies and sensitivities | Examines whether delayed reactions to foods may contribute to inflammation or other health issues. Offered by US BioTek Laboratories, Metametrix Clinical Laboratory, and ELISA/ACT Biotechnologies. |
| --- | --- |
| **Type of Test** | **Purpose** |
| Estrogen metabolite testing: 2:16 ratio | Measures the ratio of 2-hydroxyestrone to 16α-hydroxyestrone through urine. The ratio can provide an indicator of risk for estrogen-sensitive cancers. Offered by Metametrix Clinical Laboratory and Meridian Valley Lab. |
| Iodine loading test | Examines whether there is a sufficient level of iodine. A 50-milligram dose is ingested, and urine is collected for twenty-four hours and examined to see the level of excretion. This helps to determine how much, if any, supplementation is required. Offered by Vitamin Research Products and Labrix Clinical Services. |

# Retreats

*Casting for Recovery*
**castingforrecovery.org**
Free fly-fishing weekend retreat for women who have or have had breast cancer.

*Commonweal*
**www.commonweal.org**
A weeklong integrated program featuring massage, meditation, and more.

*Harmony Hill Retreat Center*
**harmonyhill.org**
Free cancer programs in Washington state for patients and their families.

### Healing Odyssey
**healingodyssey.org**

Lake Forest, California, weekend retreats for women cancer survivors.

### Hilltop Retreat
507-288-8354

Mayo Clinic–sponsored spiritual weekend retreat.

### Kokolulu Farm and Cancer Retreats
**cancer-retreats.org**

Free cancer retreats in Hawaii for patients and a guest.

### Life Choices Wellness Center
800-439-0083

A retreat center in Saluda, North Carolina, offering one-week retreats on a sliding scale of rates.

### Mending in the Mountains
406-388-4988

Women's cancer-survivor retreat at the Lone Mountain Ranch in Big Sky, Montana.

### Smith Center for Healing and the Arts
**www.smithfarm.com**

A wellness center in Washington, DC, that offers extended weekend retreats focusing on healing and the arts.

### Stowe Weekend of Hope
**stowehope.org**
800-GO-STOWE

One weekend each spring, the town of Stowe, Vermont, opens its fifty-five hotels and lodges to cancer survivors and their families at no charge. Amtrak provides a limited number of free seats for survivors to get to Stowe from Washington, DC.

### Wind River Cancer Wellness Retreats and Programs
**www.windriverservices.org**

Free cancer wellness retreat in North Carolina.

# REFERENCES

Abramson, J. L., and V. Vaccarino. 2002. "Relationship between Physical Activity and Inflammation among Apparently Healthy Middle-Aged and Older US Adults." *Archives of Internal Medicine* 162 (11):1286–92.

Aceves, C., B. Anguiano, and G. J. Delgado. 2005. "Is Iodine a Gatekeeper of the Integrity of the Mammary Gland?" *Journal of Mammary Gland Biology and Neoplasia* 10 (2):189–96.

Adams, L. S., Y. Zhang, N. P. Seeram, D. Heber, and S. Chen. 2010. "Pomegranate Ellagitannin–Derived Compounds Exhibit Antiproliferative and Antiaromatase Activity in Breast Cancer Cells in Vitro." *Cancer Prevention Research* 3 (1):108–13. doi:10.1158/1940-6207.CAPR-08-0225.

Adlercreutz, H., T. Fotsis, C. Bannwart, K. Wähälä, T. Mäkelä, G. Brunow, and T. Hase. 1986. "Determination of Urinary Lignans and Phytoestrogen Metabolites, Potential Antiestrogens and Anticarcinogens, in Urine of Women on Various Habitual Diets." *Journal of Steroid Biochemistry and Molecular Biology* 25 (5B):791–97.

Aggarwal, B. B., H. Ichikawa, P. Garodia, P. Weerasinghe, G. Sethi, I. D. Bhatt, M. K. Pandey, S. Shishodia, and M. G. Nair. 2006. "From Traditional Ayurvedic Medicine to Modern Medicine: Identification of Therapeutic Targets for Suppression of Inflammation and Cancer." *Expert Opinion on Therapeutic Targets* 10 (1):87–118. doi:10.1517/14728222.10.1.87.

Aggarwall, B. B., S. Shishodia, Y. Takada, S. Banerjee, R. A. Newman, C. E. Bueso-Ramos, and J. E. Price. 2005. "Curcumin Suppresses the Paclitaxel-Induced Nuclear Factor-κB Pathway in Breast Cancer Cells and Inhibits Lung

Metastasis of Human Breast Cancer in Nude Mice." *Clinical Cancer Research* 11 (20):7490–98.

Ahuja, K. D., I. K. Robertson, D. P. Geraghty, and M. J. Ball. 2006. "Effects of Chili Consumption on Postprandial Glucose, Insulin, and Energy Metabolism." *American Journal of Clinical Nutrition* 84 (1):63–69.

Aleksandrowicz, J., J. Blicharski, A. Dzigwska, and J. Lisiewicz. 1970. "Leuko- and Oncogenesis in the Light of Studies on the Metabolism of Magnesium and Its Turnover in Biocenosis." *Acta Medica Polona* 11 (4):289–302.

Allred, C. D., K. F. Allred, Y. H. Ju, T. S. Goeppinger, D. R. Doerge, and W. C. Helferich. 2004. "Soy Processing Influences Growth of Estrogen-Dependent Breast Cancer Tumors." *Carcinogenesis* 25 (9):1649–57. doi:10.1093/carcin/bgh178.

Althuis, M. D., D. R. Brogan, R. J. Coates, J. R. Daling, M. D. Gammon, K. E. Malone, J. B. Schoenberg, and L. A. Brinton. 2003. "Hormonal Content and Potency of Oral Contraceptives and Breast Cancer Risk among Young Women." *British Journal of Cancer* 88 (1):50–57.

American Cancer Society (ACS). 2010a. "DES Exposure: Questions and Answers." www.cancer.org/docroot/CRI/content/CRI_2_6x_DES_Exposure _Questions_and_Answers.asp. (accessed November 5, 2010).

———. 2010b. "Diet and Physical Activity: What's the Cancer Connection?" www.cancer.org/Cancer/CancerCauses/DietandPhysicalActivity/diet-and -physical-activity (accessed November 4, 2010).

———. 2010c. "Soybean." www.cancer.org/Treatment/TreatmentandSide Effects/ComplementaryandAlternativeMedicine/DietandNutrition/soybean (accessed November 20, 2010).

———. 2011a. "ACS Guidelines on Nutrition and Physical Activity for Cancer Prevention." www.cancer.org/Healthy/EatHealthyGetActive/ACSGuidelines onNutritionPhysicalActivityforCancerPrevention/acs-guidelines-on -nutrition-and-physical-activity-for-cancer-prevention-activity (accessed August 30, 2011).

———. 2011b. "What Are the Risk Factors for Breast Cancer?" www.cancer .org/cancer/breastcancer/detailedguide/breast-cancer-risk-factors (accessed November 5, 2010).

American Institute for Cancer Research (AICR). 2007. *Food, Nutrition, Physical Activity, and the Prevention of Cancer: A Global Perspective.* Washington, DC: World Cancer Research Fund and American Institute for Cancer Research.

Ames, B. N. 2006. "Low Micronutrient Intake May Accelerate the Degenerative Diseases of Aging through Allocation of Scarce Micronutrients by Triage." *Proceedings of the National Academy of Sciences* 103 (47):17589–94.

Anbar, M. 1994. *"Quantitative Dynamic Telethermometry in Medical Diagnosis and Management."* Boca Raton, FL: CRC Press.

Anton, S. D., C. K. Martin, H. Han, S. Coulon, W. T. Cefalu, P. Geiselman, and D. A. Williamson. 2010. "Effects of Stevia, Aspartame, and Sucrose on Food Intake, Satiety, and Postprandial Glucose and Insulin Levels." *Appetite* 55 (1):37–43.

Arunabh, S., S. Pollack, J. Yeh, and J. F. Aloia. 2003. "Body Fat Content and 25-Hydroxyvitamin D Levels in Healthy Women." *Journal of Clinical Endocrinology and Metabolism* 88 (1):157–61.

Aschengrau, A., S. Rogers, and D. Ozonoff. 2003. "Perchloroethylene-Contaminated Drinking Water and the Risk of Breast Cancer: Additional Results from Cape Cod, Massachusetts, USA." *Environmental Health Perspectives* 111 (2):167–73.

Bachmeier, B. E., I. V. Mohrenz, V. Mirisola, E. Schleicher, F. Romeo, C. Höhneke, M. Jochum, A. G. Nerlich, and U. Pfeffer. 2008. "Curcumin Downregulates the Inflammatory Cytokines CXCL1 and -2 in Breast Cancer Cells via NFκB." *Carcinogenesis* 29 (4):779–89. doi:10.1093/carcin/bgm248.

Bachmeier, B., A. G. Nerlich, C. M. Iancu, M. Cilli, E. Schleicher, R. Vené, R. Dell'Eva, M. Jochum, A. Albini, and U. Pfeffer. 2007. "The Chemopreventive Polyphenol Curcumin Prevents Hematogenous Breast Cancer Metastases in Immunodeficient Mice." *Cellular Physiology and Biochemistry* 19 (1–4):137–52.

Balch, J. F., and P. A. Balch. 1997. *Prescription for Nutritional Healing.* 2nd ed. New York: Avery Publishing Group.

Bauman, E. 2009. "Nutritional Supplements: Can't Live with Them, Can't Live without Them." In *Nutrition Educator Handbook*, 424–34. Penngrove, CA: Bauman College.

Bergner, P. 1996. *The Healing Power of Garlic: The Enlightened Person's Guide to Nature's Most Versatile Medicinal Plant.* Rocklin, CA: Prima Publishing.

Berkson, D. L. 2000. *Hormone Deception: How Everyday Foods and Products Are Disrupting Your Hormones—and How to Protect Yourself and Your Family.* Chicago: Contemporary Books.

Bland, J. 2010. "Confronting Cancer as a Chronic Disease: Primary Care Takes a 360-Degree View," 17th International Symposium on Functional Medicine, May 20–23, Carlsbad, CA.

Blaylock, R. L. 2003. *Natural Strategies for Cancer Patients.* New York: Kensington Publishing.

Block, K. I. 2009. *Life Over Cancer: The Block Center Program for Integrative Cancer Treatment.* New York: Bantam Books.

Bluming, A. Z., and C. Tavris. 2009. "Hormone Replacement Therapy: Real Concerns and False Alarms." *Cancer Journal* 15 (2):93–104.

Boccardo, F., M. Puntoni, P. Guglielmini, and A. Rubagotti. 2006. "Enterolactone as a Risk Factor for Breast Cancer: A Review of the Published Evidence." *Clinica chimica acta* 365 (1–2):58–67.

Bohlooly-Y M., B. Olsson, C. E. Bruder, D. Lindén, K. Sjögren, M. Bjursell, E. Egecioglu, L. Svensson, P. Brodin, J. C. Waterton, O. G. Isaksson, F. Sundler, B. Ahrén, C. Ohlsson, J. Oscarsson, and J. Törnell. 2005. "Growth Hormone Overexpression in the Central Nervous System Results in Hyperphagia-Induced Obesity Associated with Insulin Resistance and Dyslipidemia." *Diabetes* 54 (1):51–62.

Bounous, G., P. Kongshavn, and P. Gold. 1988. "The Immunoenhancing Property of Dietary Whey Protein Concentrate." *Clinical and Investigative Medicine* 11 (4):271–78.

Boyd, B. 2010. "Folic Acid and Cancer: The Folic Acid / Folate Controversy." Clinical Rounds web seminar, August 18. Suffield, CT: Designs for Health.

Brem, S. S., D. Zagzag, A. M. Tsanaclis, S. Gately, M. P. Elkouby, and S. E. Brien. 1990. "Inhibition of Angiogenesis and Tumor Growth in the Brain: Suppression of Endothelial Cell Turnover by Penicillamine and the Depletion of Copper, an Angiogenic Cofactor." *American Journal of Pathology* 137 (5):1121–42.

Bianchini, F., R. Kaaks, and H. Vainio. 2002. "Overweight, Obesity, and Cancer Risk." *Lancet Oncology* 3 (9):565–74.

Brody, J. G., K. B. Moysich, O. Humblet, K. R. Attfield, G. P. Beehler, and R. A. Rudel. 2007. "Environmental Pollutants and Breast Cancer: Epidemiologic Studies." *Cancer* 109 (Suppl. 12):2667–711.

Brownstein, D. 2008. *Iodine: Why You Need It, Why You Can't Live without It.* 3rd ed. West Bloomfield, MI: Medical Alternatives Press.

Caldwell, K. L., G. A. Miller, R. Y. Wang, R. B. Jain, and R. L. Jones. 2008. "Iodine Status of the U.S. Population, National Health and Nutrition Examination Survey 2003–2004." *Thyroid* 18 (11):1207–14.

Cameron, E., and L. Pauling. 1976. "Supplemental Ascorbate in the Supportive Treatment of Cancer: Prolongation of Survival Times in Terminal Human Cancer." *Proceedings of the National Academy of Sciences* 73 (10):3685–89.

Campbell, K. L., and A. McTiernan. 2007. "Exercise and Biomarkers for Cancer Prevention Studies." *Journal of Nutrition* 137 (Suppl. 1):161S–69.

Carson, R. 1962. *Silent Spring.* Boston: Houghton Mifflin.

Center for Food Safety. 2011. "Genetically Engineered Crops." Washington, DC: Center for Food Safety. http.centerforfoodsafety.org/campaign/genetically-engineered-food/crops (accessed September 2, 2011).

Centers for Disease Control and Prevention (CDC). 2009. "National Report on Human Exposure to Environmental Chemicals." www.cdc.gov/exposure report (accessed October 7, 2010).

Chen, Q., L. L. Y. Chan, and E. T. S. Li. 2003. "Bitter Melon (*Momordica charantia*) Reduces Adiposity, Lowers Serum Insulin, and Normalizes Glucose Tolerance in Rats Fed a High Fat Diet." *Journal of Nutrition* 133:1088–93.

Chlebowski, R. T., E. Aiello, and A. McTiernan. 2002. "Weight Loss in Breast Cancer Patient Management." *Journal of Clinical Oncology* 20 (4):1128–43.

Colborn, T., D. Dumanoski, and J. Peterson Myers. 1996. *Our Stolen Future: Are We Threatening Our Fertility, Intelligence, and Survival? A Scientific Detective Story.* New York: Penguin Group.

Combs Jr., G. F., and J. Lü. 2006. "Selenium as a Cancer Preventive Agent." In *Selenium: Its Molecular Biology and Role in Human Health*, edited by D. L. Hatfield, M. J. Berry, and V. N. Gladyshev, 249–64. New York: Springer Science+Business Media.

Cooke, R. 2001. *Dr. Folkman's War: Angiogenesis and the Struggle to Defeat Cancer.* 1st ed. New York: Random House.

Coussens, L. M., and Z. Werb. 2002. "Inflammation and Cancer." *Nature* 420 (6917):860–67.

Crinnion, W. J. 2000. "Environmental Medicine, Part 4: Pesticides—Biologically Persistent and Ubiquitous Toxins." *Alternative Medicine Review* 5 (5):432–47.

Crook, W. G. 1988. *Detecting Your Hidden Allergies.* Jackson, TN: Professional Books.

Cui, Y., A. B. Miller, and T. E. Rohan. 2006. "Cigarette Smoking and Breast Cancer Risk: Update of a Prospective Cohort Study." *Breast Cancer Research and Treatment* 100 (3):293–99.

Daniel, K. T. 2005. *The Whole Soy Story: The Dark Side of America's Favorite Health Food.* Washington, DC: New Trends Publishing.

Demers, A., P. Ayotte, J. Brisson, S. Dodin, J. Robert, and E. Dewailly. 2009. "Risk and Aggressiveness of Breast Cancer in Relation to Plasma Organochlorine Concentrations." *Cancer Epidemiology, Biomarkers & Prevention* February 9: 161.

Dimri, M., P. V. Bommi, A. A. Sahasrabuddhe, J. D. Kandekar, and G. P. Dimri. 2010. "Dietary Omega-3 Polyunsaturated Fatty Acids Suppress Expression of EZH2 in Breast Cancer Cells." *Carcinogenesis* 31 (3):489–95. doi:10.1093 /carcin/bgp305.

Dolecek, T. A., B. J. McCarthy, C. E. Joslin, C. E. Peterson, S. Kim, S. A. Freels, and F. G. Davis. 2010. "Prediagnosis Food Patterns Are Associated with Length of Survival from Epithelial Ovarian Cancer." *Journal of the American Dietetic Association* 110 (3):369–82.

Dufault, R., B. LeBlanc, R. Schnoll, C. Cornett, L. Schweitzer, D. Wallinga, J. Hightower, L. Patrick, and W. J. Lukiw. 2009. "Mercury from Chlor-Alkali Plants: Measured Concentrations in Food Product Sugar." *Environmental Health* 8:2. doi:10.1186/1476-069X-8-2.

Durlach, J., M. Bara, A. Guiet-Bara, and P. Collery. 1986. "Relationship between Magnesium, Cancer, and Carcinogenic or Anticancer Metals." *Anticancer Research* 6 (6):1353–61.

El-Bayoumy, K., R. Sinha, J. T. Pinto, and R. S. Rivlin. 2006. "Cancer Chemoprevention by Garlic and Garlic-Containing Sulfur and Selenium Compounds." *Journal of Nutrition* 136 (Suppl. 3):864S–69S.

Eliassen, A. H., S. A. Missmer, S. S. Tworoger, and S. E. Hankinson. 2008. "Circulating 2-Hydroxy and 16α-Hydroxy Estrone Levels and Risk of Breast Cancer among Postmenopausal Women." *Cancer Epidemiology, Biomarkers, and Prevention* 17:2029–35. doi:10.1158/1055-9965.EPI-08-0262.

Environmental Working Group (EWG). 2007. "EWG Research: A Survey of Bisphenol A in U.S. Canned Foods," March 5, Washington DC. www.ewg .org/reports/bisphenola (accessed April 22, 2011).

———. 2009. "National Drinking Water Database: Full Report." Washington DC. http.ewg.org/tap-water/rating-big-city-water (accessed April 16, 2011).

———. 2010. "New Study Confirms BPA Exposures from Receipts: New Study Confirms BPA in Receipts—Green Chemistry Pioneer's Paper Documents Risk." Washington, DC. www.ewg.org/book/export/html/28608 (accessed August 30, 2011).

Epstein, S. S. 1996. "Unlabeled Milk from Cows Treated with Biosynthetic Growth Hormones: A Case of Regulatory Abdication." *International Journal of Health Services* 26 (1):173–85.

———. 2009. *Toxic Beauty: How Cosmetics and Personal Care Products Endanger Your Health…and What You Can Do about It.* With R. Fitzgerald. Dallas, TX: BenBella Books.

Eskin, B. A., D. G. Bartuska, M. R. Dunn, G. Jacob, and M. B. Dratman. 1967. "Mammary Gland Dysplasia in Iodine Deficiency: Studies in Rats." *Journal of the American Medical Association* 200 (8):691–95. doi:10.1001/jama.1967 .03120210077014.

Esmaillzadeh, A., M. Kimiagar, Y. Mehrabi, L. Azadbakht, F. B. Hu, and W. C. Willett. 2006. "Fruit and Vegetable Intakes, C-Reactive Protein, and the Metabolic Syndrome." *American Journal of Clinical Nutrition* 84 (6):1489–97.

EU Council Directive. 1976. Council Directive 76/768/EEC of 27 July 1976 on the approximation of the laws of the Member States relating to cosmetic products. European Commission Consumer Affairs.

———. 2005. Directive 2005/84/EC of the European Parliament and of the Council of 14 December 2005 amending for the 22nd time Council Directive 76/769/EEC on the approximation of the laws, regulations, and administrative provisions of the Member States relating to restrictions on the marketing and use of certain dangerous substances and preparations (phthalates in toys and childcare articles). Official Journal of the European Union.

Fallon, S. 2001. *Nourishing Traditions.* With M. G. Enig. Rev. 2nd ed. Washington, DC: New Trends Publishing.

Fasano, A., I. Berti, T. Gerarduzzi, T. Not, R. B. Colletti, S. Drago, Y. Elitsur, P. H. R. Green, S. Guandalini, I. D. Hill, M. Pietzak, A. Ventura, M. Thorpe, D. Kryszak, F. Fornaroli, S. S. Wasserman, J. A. Murray, and K. Horvath. 2003. "Prevalence of Celiac Disease in At-Risk and Not-At-Risk Groups in the United States: A Large Multicenter Study." *Archives of Internal Medicine* 163 (3):286–92.

Fidelus, R. K., and M. F. Tsan. 1986. "Enhancement of Intracellular Glutathione Promotes Lymphocyte Activation by Mitogen." *Cellular Immunology*. 97 (1): 155–63. doi:10.1016/0008-8749(86)90385-0.

Fishman, J., L. Hellman, B. Zumoff, and T. F. Gallagher. 1965. "Effect of Thyroid on Hydroxylation of Estrogen in Man." *Journal of Clinical Endocrinology and Metabolism* 25 (3):365–68. doi:10.1210/jcem-25-3-365.

Flavin, D. F. 2007. "A Lipoxygenase Inhibitor in Breast Cancer Brain Metastases." *Journal of Neuro-Oncology* 82 (1):91–93. doi:10.1007/s11060-006-9248-4.

Frassetto, L. A., K. M. Todd, R. C. Morris Jr., and A. Sebastian. 2000. "Worldwide Incidence of Hip Fracture in Elderly Women: Relation to Consumption of Animal and Vegetable Foods." *Journals of Gerontology* 55 (10):M585–92.

Fung, T. T., F. B. Hu, M. A. Pereira, S. Liu, M. J. Stampfer, G. A. Colditz, and W. C. Willett. 2002. "Whole-Grain Intake and the Risk of Type 2 Diabetes: A Prospective Study in Men." *American Journal of Clinical Nutrition* 76 (3): 535–40.

Gaikwad, N. W., L. Yang, P. Muti, J. L. Meza, S. Pruthi, J. N. Ingle, E. G. Rogan, and E. L. Cavalieri. 2008. "The Molecular Etiology of Breast Cancer: Evidence from Biomarkers of Risk." *International Journal of Cancer* 122 (9):1949–57.

Gamet-Payrastre, L., P. Li, S. Lumeau, G. Cassar, M.-A. Dupont, S. Chevolleau, N. Gasc, J. Tulliez, and F. Tercé. 2000. "Sulforaphane, a Naturally Occurring Isothiocyanate, Induces Cell Cycle Arrest and Apoptosis in HT29 Human Colon Cancer Cells." *Cancer Research* 60 (5):1426–33.

Gao, X., Y. X. Xu, N. Janakiraman, R. A. Chapman, and S. C. Gautam. 2001. "Immunomodulatory Activity of Resveratrol: Suppression of Lymphocyte Proliferation, Development of Cell-Mediated Cytotoxicity, and Cytokine Production." *Biochemical Pharmacology* 62 (9):1299–308.

Garg, A. 1998. "High-Monounsaturated-Fat Diets for Patients with Diabetes Mellitus: A Meta-Analysis." *American Journal of Clinical Nutrition* 67 (Suppl. 3):577S–82.

Garland, C. F., F. C. Garland, E. D. Gorham, M. Lipkin, H. Newmark, S. B. Mohr, and M. F. Holick. 2006. "Dealing with Innovation and Uncertainty: The Role of Vitamin D in Cancer Prevention." *American Journal of Public Health* 96 (2):252–61. doi:10.2105/AJPH.2004.045260.

Garland, C. F., E. D. Gorham, S. B. Mohr, W. B. Grant, E. L. Giovannucci, M. Lipkin, H. Newmark, M. F. Holick, and F. C. Garland. 2007. "Vitamin D and

Prevention of Breast Cancer: Pooled Analysis." *Journal of Steroid Biochemistry and Molecular Biology* 103 (3–5):708–11.

Gatenby, R. A., K. Smallbone, P. K. Maini, F. Rose, J. Averill, R. B. Nagle, L. Worrall, and R. J. Gillies. 2007. "Cellular Adaptations to Hypoxia and Acidosis during Somatic Evolution of Breast Cancer." *British Journal of Cancer* 97 (5):646–53. doi:10.1038/sj.bjc.6603922.

Gautherie, M., P. Haehnel, J. P. Walter, and L. Keith. 1982. "Long-Term Assessment of Breast Cancer Risk by Liquid-Crystal Thermal Imaging." *Progress in Clinical and Biological Research* 107:279–301.

Gershon, M. D. 1998. *The Second Brain: A Groundbreaking New Understanding of the Stomach and Intestine.* New York: HarperCollins Publishers.

Gittleman, A. L. 2008. *Get the Sugar Out: 501 Simple Ways to Cut the Sugar Out of Any Diet.* 2nd ed. New York: Three Rivers Press.

Grady, D. 2010. "First Signs of Puberty Seen in Younger Girls." *New York Times,* August 9, Research section.

Gribel, N. V., and V. G. Pashinski. 1986. "Antimetastatic Properties of Aloe Juice." [In Russian.] *Voprosy Onkologii* 32 (12):38–40.

Grinder-Pedersen, L., S. E. Rasmussen, S. Bügel, L. V. Jørgensen, L. O. Dragsted, V. Gundersen, and B. Sandström. 2003. "Effect of Diets Based on Foods from Conventional versus Organic Production on Intake and Excretion of Flavonoids and Markers of Antioxidative Defense in Humans." *Journal of Agricultural and Food Chemistry* 51 (19):5671–76. doi:10.1021/jf030217n.

Grzanna, R., L. Lindmark, and C. G. Frondoza. 2005. "Ginger: An Herbal Medicinal Product with Broad Anti-Inflammatory Actions." *Journal of Medicinal Food* 8 (2):125–32.

Guarner, F., and J. R. Malagelada. 2003. "Gut Flora in Health and Disease." *Lancet* 361 (9356):512–19.

Gunter, M. J., D. R. Hoover, H. Yu, S. Wassertheil-Smoller, T. E. Rohan, J. E. Manson, J. Li, G. Y. Ho, X. Xue, G. L. Anderson, R. C. Kaplan, T. G. Harris, B. V. Howard, J. Wylie-Rosett, R. D. Burk, and H. D. Strickler. 2009. "Insulin, Insulin-Like Growth Factor-1, and Risk of Breast Cancer in Postmenopausal Women." *Journal of the National Cancer Institute* 101 (1):48–60.

Hadsell, D. L., and S. G. Bonnette. 2000. "IGF and Insulin Action in the Mammary Gland: Lessons from Transgenic and Knockout Models." *Journal of Mammary Gland Biology and Neoplasia* 5 (1):19–30. doi:10.1023/A :1009559014703.

Hankinson, S. E., W. C. Willett, G. A. Colditz, D. J. Hunter, D. S. Michaud, B. Deroo, B. Rosner, F. E. Speizer, and M. Pollak. 1998. "Circulating Concentrations of Insulin-Like Growth Factor-1 and Risk of Breast Cancer." *Lancet* 351 (9113):1393–96.

Hernandez-Reif, M., T. Field, G. Ironson, J. Beutler, Y. Vera, J. Hurley, M. A. Fletcher, S. Schanberg, C. Kuhn, and M. Fraser. 2005. "Natural Killer Cells and Lymphocytes Increase in Women with Breast Cancer Following Massage Therapy." *International Journal of Neuroscience* 115 (4):495–510. doi:10.1080 /00207450590523080.

Heustad, A. 2004. "The Amazing Health Benefits of Drinking Lemon Water." *Idaho Observer*, July.

Holick, M. F. 2004. "Vitamin D: Importance in the Prevention of Cancers, Type 1 Diabetes, Heart Disease, and Osteoporosis." *American Journal of Clinical Nutrition* 79 (3):362–71.

Holliday, J. C., and M. P. Cleaver. 2008. "Medicinal Value of the Caterpillar Fungi Species of the Genus *Cordyceps* (Fr.) Link (Ascomycetes): A Review." *International Journal of Medicinal Mushrooms* 10 (3):219–34. doi:10.1615/Int JMedMushr.v10.i3.30.

Hong, S. A., K. Kim, S. J. Nam, G. Kong, and M. K. Kim. 2008. "A Case-Control Study on the Dietary Intake of Mushrooms and Breast Cancer Risk among Korean Women." *International Journal of Cancer* 122 (4):919–23.

Howenstine, J. A. 2008. *A Physician's Guide to Natural Health Products That Work.* 2nd ed. Miami, FL: Penhurst Books.

Høyer, A. P., P. Grandjean, T. Jørgensen, J. W. Brock, and H. B. Hartvig. 1998. "Organochlorine Exposure and Risk of Breast Cancer." *Lancet* 352 (9143): 1816–20.

Hughes, D., and J. Hughes. 2006. "Mind-Body Medicine and the Future of Holistic Health Care: An Interview with Dr. Bernie Siegel." *Share Guide* March to April (84):16

Hunt, B. J., and L. F. Belanger. 1972. "Localized, Multiform, Sub-periosteal Hyperplasia and Generalized Osteomyelosclerosis in Magnesium-Deficient Rats." *Calcified Tissue Research* 9 (1):17–27.

Hyman, M. A. 2007. "The Life Cycles of Women: Restoring Balance." *Alternative Therapies* 13 (3):10–16.

Iwasaki, M., M. Inoue, T. Otani, S. Sasazuki, N. Kurahashi, T. Miura, S. Yamamoto, and S. Tsugane. 2008. "Plasma Isoflavone Level and Subsequent Risk of Breast Cancer among Japanese Women: A Nested Case-Control Study from the Japan Public Health Center–Based Prospective Study Group." *Journal of Clinical Oncology* 26 (10):1677–83. doi:10.1200/JCO.2007.13.9964.

Jackson, J. R., M. P. Seed, C. H. Kircher, D. A. Willoughby, and J. D. Winkler. 1997. "The Codependence of Angiogenesis and Chronic Inflammation." *FASEB Journal* 11 (6):457–65.

Jarvill-Taylor, K. J., R. A. Anderson, and D. J. Graves. 2001. "A Hydroxychalcone Derived from Cinnamon Functions as a Mimetic for Insulin in 3T3-L1 Adipocytes." *Journal of the American College of Nutrition* 20 (4):327–36.

Jarvis, D. C. 1958. *Folk Medicine: A Vermont Doctor's Guide to Good Health*. New York: Henry Holt and Company.

Jefcoate, C. R., J. G. Liehr, R. J. Santen, T. R. Sutter, J. D. Yager, W. Yue, S. J. Santner, R. Tekmal, L. Demers, R. Pauley, F. Naftolin, G. Mor, and L. Berstein. 2000. "Tissue-Specific Synthesis and Oxidative Metabolism of Estrogens." *Journal of the National Cancer Institute Monographs* 27:95–112.

Jerry, D. J. 2007. "Roles for Estrogen and Progesterone in Breast Cancer Prevention." *Breast Cancer Research* 9 (2):102.

John, E. M., G. G. Schwartz, D. M. Dreon, and J. Koo. 1999. "Vitamin D and Breast Cancer Risk: The NHANES I Epidemiologic Follow-Up Study, 1971–1975 to 1992." *Cancer Epidemiology, Biomarkers, and Prevention* 8 (5): 399–406.

Ju, Y. H., D. R. Doerge, K. F. Allred, C. D. Allred, and W. G. Helferich. 2002. "Dietary Genistein Negates the Inhibitory Effect of Tamoxifen on Growth of Estrogen-Dependent Human Breast Cancer (MCF-7) Cells Implanted in Athymic Mice." *Cancer Research* 62 (9):2474–77.

Kabat, G. C., E. S. O'Leary, M. D. Gammon, D. W. Sepkovic, S. L. Teitelbaum, J. A. Britton, M. B. Terry, A. I. Neugut, and H. L. Bradlow. 2006. "Estrogen Metabolism and Breast Cancer." *Epidemiology* 17 (1):80–88.

Kawa, J. M., C. G. Taylor, and R. Przybylski. 2003. "Buckwheat Concentrate Reduces Serum Glucose in Streptozotocin-Diabetic Rats." *Journal of Agricultural and Food Chemistry* 51 (25):7287–91. doi:10.1021/jf0302153.

Kawamura, T., and T. Sobue. 2005. "Comparison of Breast Cancer Mortality in Five Countries: France, Italy, Japan, the UK, and the USA, from the WHO Mortality Database (1960–2000)." *Japanese Journal of Clinical Oncology* 35 (12):758–59.

Kelleher, S. L., Y. A. Seo, and V. Lopez. 2009. "Mammary Gland Zinc Metabolism: Regulation and Dysregulation." *Genes and Nutrition* 4 (2):83–94. doi:10.1007/s12263-009-0119-4.

Kim, M. K., and J. H. Y. Park. 2009. "Cruciferous Vegetable Intake and the Risk of Human Cancer: Epidemiological Evidence." *Proceedings of the Nutrition Society* 68:103–10. doi:10.1017/S0029665108008884.

King, D. E., A. G. Mainous III, M. E. Geesey, B. M. Egan, and S. Rehman. 2006. "Magnesium Supplement Intake and C-Reactive Protein Levels in Adults." *Nutrition Research* 26 (5):193–96. doi:10.1016/j.nutres.2006.05.001.

Kobori, M., M. Ohnishi-Kameyama, Y. Akimoto, C. Yukizaki, and M. Yoshida. 2008. "α-Eleostearic Acid and Its Dihydroxy Derivative Are Major Apoptosis-Inducing Components of Bitter Gourd." *Journal of Agricultural and Food Chemistry* 56 (22):10515–20. doi:10.1021/jf8020877.

Krishnan, A. V., S. Swami, L. Peng, J. Wang, J. Moreno, and D. Feldman. 2010. "Tissue-Selective Regulation of Aromatase Expression by Calcitriol: Implications for Breast Cancer Therapy." *Endocrinology* 151 (1):32–42.

Kumar, S. N., U. V. Mani, and I. Mani. 2010. "An Open Label Study on the Supplementation of *Gymnema sylvestre* in Type 2 Diabetics." *Journal of Dietary Supplements* 7 (3):273–82.

Lahmann, P. H., L. Lissner, and G. Berglund. 2004. "Breast Cancer Risk in Overweight Postmenopausal Women." *Cancer Epidemiology, Biomarkers, and Prevention* 13 (8):1414.

Lapidot, T., M. D. Walker, and J. Kanner. 2002. "Can Apple Antioxidants Inhibit Tumor Cell Proliferation? Generation of H2O2 during Interaction of Phenolic Compounds with Cell Culture Media." *Journal of Agricultural and Food Chemistry* 50 (11):3156–60. doi:10.1021/jf011522g.

Larsson, S. C., L. Bergkvist, and A. Wolk. 2009. "Glycemic Load, Glycemic Index, and Breast Cancer Risk in a Prospective Cohort of Swedish Women." *International Journal of Cancer* 125 (1):153–57.

Lau, B. 1988. *Garlic for Health.* Twin Lakes, WI: Lotus Press.

Lee, J. R. 2001. *Natural Progesterone: The Multiple Roles of a Remarkable Hormone.* 2nd ed. Oxfordshire, UK: Jon Carpenter Publishing.

Leffall Jr., L. D., and M. L. Kripke (The President's Cancer Panel). 2010. *2008–2009 Annual Report, President's Cancer Panel: Reducing Environmental Cancer Risk—What We Can Do Now.* With S. H. Reuben. Bethesda, MD: US Department of Health and Human Services, National Institutes of Health, and National Cancer Institute.

Lei, X. Y., S. Q. Yao, X. Y. Zu, Z. X. Huang, L. J. Liu, M. Zhong, B. Y. Zhu, S. S. Tang, and D. F. Liao. 2008. "Apoptosis Induced by Diallyl Disulfide in Human Breast Cancer Cell Line MCF-7." *Acta Pharmacologica Sinica* 29 (10):1233–39. doi:10.1111/j.1745-7254.2008.00851.x.

Lemaire, I., V. Assinewe, P. Cano, D. V. Awang, and J. T. Arnason. 1999. "Stimulation of Interleukin-1 and -6 Production in Alveolar Macrophages by the Neotropical Liana, Uncaria tomentosa (Uña de Gato)." *Journal of Ethnopharmacology* 64 (2):109–15.

Lemon, H. M., H. H. Wotiz, L. Parsons, and P. J. Mozden. 1966. "Reduced Estriol Excretion in Patients with Breast Cancer Prior to Endocrine Therapy." *Journal of the American Medical Association* 196 (13):1128–36. doi:10.1001/jama.1966.03100260066020.

Liao, Y., X. Du, and B. Lönnerdal. 2010. "miR-214 Regulates Lactoferrin Expression and Pro-Apoptotic Function in Mammary Epithelial Cells." *Journal of Nutrition* 140 (9):1552–56. doi:10.3945/jn.110.124289.

Lipski, E. 2005. *Digestive Wellness.* 3rd ed. New York: McGraw-Hill.

Liu, M., T. Sakamaki, M. C. Casimiro, N. E. Willmarth, A. A. Quong, X. Ju, J. Ojeifo, X. Jiao, W. S. Yeow, S. Katiyar, L. A. Shirley, D. Joyce, M. P. Lisanti, C. Albanese, and R. G. Pestel. 2010. "The Canonical NF-κB Pathway Governs Mammary Tumorigenesis in Transgenic Mice and Tumor Stem Cell Expansion." *Cancer Research* 70 (24):10464–73. doi:10.1158/0008-5472.CAN -10-0732.

Liu, R. H. 2004. "Potential Synergy of Phytochemicals in Cancer Prevention: Mechanism of Action." *Journal of Nutrition* 134 (Suppl. 12):3479S–485.

Luck, S. J. 2010. "Eco Nutrition: Nutritional and Environmental Influences." Presentation at the 3rd Annual Evidence-Based Complementary and Alternative Cancer Therapies conference, January 8, West Palm Beach, FL.

MacKinnon, L. T. 2000. "Overtraining Effects on Immunity and Performance in Athletes." *Immunology and Cell Biology* 78:502–09. doi:10.1111/j.1440-1711 .2000.t01-7-.

Martin, K. R., and S. K. Brophy. 2010. "Commonly Consumed and Specialty Dietary Mushrooms Reduce Cellular Proliferation in MCF-7 Human Breast Cancer Cells." *Experimental Biology and Medicine* 235 (11):1306–14.

Maruti, S. S., C. M. Ulrich, and E. White. 2009. "Folate and One-Carbon Metabolism Nutrients from Supplements and Diet in Relation to Breast Cancer Risk." *American Journal of Clinical Nutrition* 89 (2):624–33.

Maury, E., and S. M. Brichard. 2010. "Adipokine Dysregulation, Adipose Tissue Inflammation and Metabolic Syndrome." *Molecular and Cellular Endocrinology* 314 (1):1–16.

McCann, S. E., P. Muti, D. Vito, S. B. Edge, M. Trevisan, and J. L. Freudenheim. 2004. "Dietary Lignan Intakes and Risk of Pre- and Postmenopausal Breast Cancer." *International Journal of Cancer* 111 (3):440–43.

McIntyre, A., P. R. Gibson, and G. P. Young. 1993. "Butyrate Production from Dietary Fibre and Protection against Large Bowel Cancer in a Rat Model." *Gut* 34 (3):386–91.

McTiernan, A., C. Kooperberg, E. White, S. Wilcox, R. Coates, L. L. Adams-Campbell, N. Woods, and J. Ockene. 2003. "Recreational Physical Activity and the Risk of Breast Cancer in Postmenopausal Women: The Women's Health Initiative Cohort Study." *Journal of the American Medical Association* 290 (10):1331–36.

McTiernan, A., S. S. Tworoger, C. M. Ulrich, Y. Yasui, M. L. Irwin, K. B. Rajan, B. Sorensen, R. E. Rudolph, D. Bowen, F. Z. Stanczyk, J. D. Potter, and R. S. Schwartz. 2004. "Effect of Exercise on Serum Estrogens in Postmenopausal Women: A 12-Month Randomized Clinical Trial." *Cancer Research* 64 (8):2923–28.

Meilahn, E. N., B. De Stavola, D. S. Allen, I. Fentiman, H. L. Bradlow, D. W. Sepkovic, and L. H. Kuller. 1998. "Do Urinary Oestrogen Metabolites Predict

Breast Cancer? Guernsey III Cohort Follow-Up." *British Journal of Cancer* 78 (9):1250–55.

Memon, A. R., T. G. Kazi, H. I. Afridi, M. K. Jamali, M. B. Arain, N. Jalbani, and N. Syed. 2007. "Evaluations of Zinc Status in Whole Blood and Scalp Hair of Female Cancer Patients." *Clinica Chimica Acta* 379 (1–2):66–70. doi:10.1016/j.cca.2006.12.009.

Micke, P., K. M. Beeh, and R. Buhl. 2002. "Effects of Long-Term Supplementation with Whey Proteins on Plasma Glutathione Levels of HIV-Infected Patients." *European Journal of Nutrition* 41 (1):12–18. doi:10.1007/s003940200001.

Miller, G. 2006. "Nanomaterials, Sunscreens, and Cosmetics: Small Ingredients, Big Risks." With L. Archer, E. Pica, D. Bell, R. Senjen, and G. Kimbrell. May. www.foe.org/sites/default/files/final_USA_web.pdf (accessed April 21, 2011).

Moiseeva, E. P., G. M. Almeida, G. D. Jones, and M. M. Manson. 2007. "Extended Treatment with Physiologic Concentrations of Dietary Phytochemicals Results in Altered Gene Expression, Reduced Growth, and Apoptosis of Cancer Cells." *Molecular Cancer Therapeutics* 6 (11):3071–79. doi:10.1158/1535-7163.MCT-07-0117.

Morris, R. D., A. M. Audet, I. F. Angelillo, T. C. Chalmers, and F. Mosteller. 1992. "Chlorination, Chlorination By-Products, and Cancer: A Meta-Analysis." *American Journal of Public Health* 82 (7):955–63.

Mouse Genome Sequencing Consortium. 2002. "Initial Sequencing and Comparative Analysis of the Mouse Genome." *Nature* 420 (6915):520–62.

Mozaffarian, D., T. Pischon, S. E. Hankinson, N. Rifai, K. Joshipura, W. C. Willett, and E. B. Rimm. 2004. "Dietary Intake of Trans Fatty Acids and Systemic Inflammation in Women." *American Journal of Clinical Nutrition* 79 (4):606–12.

Muñoz-de-Toro, M., M. Durando, P. M. Beldoménico, H. R. Beldoménico, L. Kass, S. R. García, and E. H. Luque. 2006. "Estrogenic Microenvironment Generated by Organochlorine Residues in Adipose Mammary Tissue Modulates Biomarker Expression in ERα-Positive Breast Carcinomas." *Breast Cancer Research* 8:R47. doi:10.1186/bcr1534.

Murray, T. J., M. V. Maffini, A. A. Ucci, C. Sonnenschein, and A. M. Soto. 2007. "Induction of Mammary Gland Ductal Hyperplasias and Carcinoma *in Situ* Following Fetal Bisphenol A Exposure." *Reproductive Toxicology* 23 (3):383–90. doi:10.1016/j.reprotox.2006.10.002.

Muti, P., H. L. Bradlow, A. Micheli, V. Krogh, J. L. Freudenheim, H. J. Schünemann, M. Stanulla, J. Yang, D. W. Sepkovic, M. Trevisan, and F. Berrino. 2000. "Estrogen Metabolism and Risk of Breast Cancer: A Prospective Study of the 2:16α-Hydroxyestrone Ratio in Premenopausal and Postmenopausal Women." *Epidemiology* 11 (6):635–40.

National Cancer Institute (NCI). 2009. "Fact Sheet: Physical Activity and Cancer." www.cancer.gov/cancertopics/factsheet/prevention/physicalactivity (accessed September 1, 2011).

———. 2010. "SEER Stat Fact Sheets: Breast." http://seer.cancer.gov/statfacts /html/breast.html (accessed November 9, 2010).

———. 2011. "Cancer Causes and Risk Factors." http.cancer.gov/cancertopics /prevention-genetics-causes/causes (accessed April 14, 2011).

National Institute of Environmental Health Sciences (NIEHS). 2010. "Since You Asked: Bisphenol A—Questions and Answers about Bisphenol A." Triangle Park, NC: NIEHS, National Institutes of Health. http.niehs.nih.gov/news /media/questions/sya-bpa.cfm (accessed October 14, 2010).

National Institutes of Health (NIH). 2002. "NHLBI Stops Trial of Estrogen Plus Progestin Due to Increased Breast Cancer Risk, Lack of Overall Benefit." http.nhlbi.nih.gov/new/press/02-07-09.htm (accessed August 27, 2011).

———. 2007. "Genetics Home Reference: Genetic Conditions—Breast Cancer." U.S. National Library of Medicine. ghr.nlm.nih.gov/condition/breast-cancer (accessed December 20, 2010).

Natural Resources Defense Council (NRDC). 2003. "Tap Water at Risk: Bush Administration Actions Endanger America's Drinking Water Supplies." In *What's on Tap? Grading Drinking Water in U.S. Cities*, 80–90. New York: NRDC.

Norikura, T., D. O. Kennedy, A. K. Nyarko, A. Kojima, I. Matsui-Yuasa. 2002. "Protective Effect of Aloe Extract against the Cytotoxicity of 1,4-naphthoquinone in Isolated Rat Hepatocytes Involves Modulations in Cellular Thiol Levels." *Pharmacology and Toxicology* 90 (5):278–84.

Ouyang, X., P. Cirillo, Y. Sautin, S. McCall, J. L. Bruchette, A. M. Diehl, R. J. Johnson, and M.F. Abdelmalek. 2008. "Fructose Consumption as a Risk Factor for Non-alcoholic Fatty Liver Disease." *Journal of Hepatology* 48 (6):993–99.

Patil, J. R., G. K. Jayaprakasha, K. N. C. Murthy, S. E. Tichy, M. B. Chetti, and B. S. Patil. 2009. "Apoptosis-Mediated Proliferation Inhibition of Human Colon Cancer Cells by Volatile Principles of *Citrus aurantifolia*." *Food Chemistry* 114 (4):1351–58.

Petersen, C. A., and M. E. Heffernan. 2008. "Serum Tumor Necrosis Factor-Alpha Concentrations Are Negatively Correlated with Serum 25(OH)D Concentrations in Healthy Women." *Journal of Inflammation* 5:10. doi:10.1186 /1476-9255-5-10.

Petrelli, J. M., E. E. Calle, C. Rodriguez, and M. J. Thun. 2002. "Body Mass Index, Height, and Postmenopausal Breast Cancer Mortality in a Prospective Cohort of US Women." *Cancer Causes and Control* 13 (4):325–32.

Pierce, B. L., R. Ballard-Barbash, L. Bernstein, R. N. Baumgartner, M. L. Neuhouser, M. H. Wener, K. B. Baumgartner, F. D. Gilliland, B. E. Sorensen,

A. McTiernan, and C. M. Ulrich. 2009. "Elevated Biomarkers of Inflammation Are Associated with Reduced Survival among Breast Cancer Patients." *Journal of Clinical Oncology* 27 (21):3437–44. doi:10.1200/JCO.2008.18.9068.

Pierce, J. P., M. L. Stefanick, S. W. Flatt, L. Natarajan, B. Sternfeld, L. Madlensky, W. K. Al-Delaimy, C. A. Thomson, S. Kealy, R. Hajek, B. A. Parker, V. A. Newman, B. Caan, and C. L. Rock. 2007. "Greater Survival after Breast Cancer in Physically Active Women with High Vegetable-Fruit Intake Regardless of Obesity." *Journal of Clinical Oncology* 25 (17):2345–51. doi:10.1200/JCO.2006.08.6819.

Pledgie-Tracy, A., M. D. Sobolewski, and N. E. Davidson. 2007. "Sulforaphane Induces Cell Type–Specific Apoptosis in Human Breast Cancer Cell Lines." *Molecular Cancer Therapeutics* 6:1013. doi:10.1158/1535-7163.MCT-06-0494.

Poulose, S. M., G. K. Jayaprakasha, R. T. Mayer, B. Girennavar, and B. S. Patil. 2007. "Purification of Citrus Limonoids and Their Differential Inhibitory Effects on Human Cytochrome P450 Enzymes." *Journal of the Science of Food and Agriculture* 87 (9):1699–1709. doi:10.1002/jsfa.2891.

Preston, B. T., I. Capellini, P. McNamara, R. A. Barton, and C. L. Nunn. 2009. "Parasite Resistance and the Adaptive Significance of Sleep." *BMC Evolutionary Biology* 9:7. doi:10.1186/1471-2148-9-7.

Quillin, P. 2005. *Beating Cancer with Nutrition.* 4th ed. With N. Quillin. Includes CD-ROM. Carlsbad, CA: Nutrition Times Press.

Ramasamy, K., and R. Agarwal. 2008. "Multitargeted Therapy of Cancer by Silymarin." *Cancer Letters* 269 (2):352–62.

Ramesha, A., N. Rao, A. R. Rao, L. N. Jannu, and S. P. Hussain. 1990. "Chemoprevention of 7,12-Dimethylbenz[α]anthracene-induced Mammary Carcinogenesis in Rat by the Combined Actions of Selenium, Magnesium, Ascorbic Acid and Retinyl Acetate." *Japanese Journal of Cancer Research* 81 (12):1239–46.

Redberg, R. F. 2009. "Cancer Risks and Radiation Exposure from Computed Tomographic Scans: How Can We Be Sure That the Benefits Outweigh the Risks?" *Archives of Internal Medicine* 169 (22):2049–50.

Rode von Essen, M., M. Kongsbak, P. Schjerling, K. Olgaard, N. Ødum, and C. Geisler. 2010. "Vitamin D Controls T Cell Antigen Receptor Signaling and Activation of Human T Cells." *Nature Immunology* 11:344–49. doi:10.1038/ni.1851.

Rossouw, J. E., G. L. Anderson, R. L. Prentice, A. Z. LaCroix, C. Kooperberg, M. L. Stefanick, R. D. Jackson, S. A. Beresford, B. V. Howard, K. C. Johnson, J. M. Kotchen, J. Ockene; Writing Group for the Women's Health Initiative Investigators. 2002. "Risks and Benefits of Estrogen plus Progestin in Healthy Postmenopausal Women: Principal Results from the Women's Health Initiative Randomized Controlled Trial." *Journal of the American Medical Association* 288 (3):321–33.

Sanchez, A. J., L. Reeser, H. S. Lau, P. Y. Yahiku, R. E. Willard, P. J. McMillan, S. Y. Cho, A. R. Magie, and U. D. Register. 1973. "Role of Sugars in Human Neutrophilic Phagocytosis." *American Journal of Clinical Nutrition* 26:1180–84.

Santisteban, G. A., J. T. Ely, E. E. Hamel, D. H. Read, and S. M. Kozawa. 1985. "Glycemic Modulation of Tumor Tolerance in a Mouse Model of Breast Cancer." *Biochemical and Biophysical Research Communications* 132 (3):1174–79.

Sardi, B. 2007. *You Don't Have to Be Afraid of Cancer Anymore: New Therapies Promise Hope and Survival.* San Dimas, CA: Here and Now Books.

Schlosser, E. 2001. *Fast Food Nation: The Dark Side of the All-American Meal.* New York: Houghton Mifflin.

Scolnik, A. J., M. C. Rubio, and R. A. Caro. 1985. "Histamine and Cancer." *Trends in Pharmacological Sciences* 6:356–57. doi:10.1016/0165-6147(85)90166-X.

Seitz, H. K., and B. Maurer. 2007. "The Relationship between Alcohol Metabolism, Estrogen Levels, and Breast Cancer Risk." *Alcohol Research and Health* 30 (1):42–43.

Selva, D. M., K. N. Hogeveen, S. M. Innis, and G. L. Hammond. 2007. "Monosaccharide-Induced Lipogenesis Regulates the Human Hepatic Sex Hormone–Binding Globulin Gene." *Journal of Clinical Investigation* 117 (12):3979–87. doi:10.1172/JCI32249.

Sgambato, A., and A. Cittadini. 2010. "Inflammation and Cancer: A Multifaceted Link." *European Review for Medical and Pharmacological Sciences* 14 (4):263–68.

Shu, X. O., Y. Zheng, H. Cai, K. Gu, Z. Chen, W. Zheng, and W. Lu. 2009. "Soy Food Intake and Breast Cancer Survival." *Journal of the American Medical Association* 302 (22):2437–43. doi:10.1001/jama.2009.1783.

Siiteri, P. K., R. I. Sholtz, P. M. Cirillo, R. D. Cohen, R. E. Christianson, B. J. van den Berg, W. R. Hopper, and B. A. Cohn. 2002. "Prospective Study of Estrogens during Pregnancy and Risk of Breast Cancer." Public Health Institute, Berkeley, CA. Abstract of presentation at Era of Hope, Department of Defense Breast Cancer Research Program Meeting, September 25–28, Orlando, FL. cdmrp.army.mil/bcrp/era/abstracts2002/p13_chemoprevention/9919358_abs.pdf (accessed August 27, 2011).

Simontacchi, C. 2000. *The Crazy Makers: How the Food Industry Is Destroying Our Brains and Harming Our Children.* New York: Jeremy P. Tarcher/Putnam.

Simopoulos, A. P. 2006. "Evolutionary Aspects of Diet, the Omega-6/Omega-3 Ratio, and Genetic Variation: Nutritional Implications for Chronic Diseases." *Biomedicine and Pharmacotherapy* 60 (9):502–7.

Smith, M. L., J. K. Lancia, T. I. Mercer, and C. Ip. 2004. "Selenium Compounds Regulate p53 by Common and Distinctive Mechanisms." *Anticancer Research* 24 (3a):1401–8.

Smith-Bindman, R., J. Lipson, R. Marcus, K.-P. Kim, M. Mahesh, R. Gould, A. Berrington de González, and D. L. Miglioretti. 2009. "Radiation Dose Associated with Common Computed Tomography Examinations and the Associated Lifetime Attributable Risk of Cancer." *Archives of Internal Medicine* 169 (22):2078–86.

Song, Z., I. Deaciuc, M. Song, D. Y. Lee, Y. Liu, X. Ji, and C. McClain. 2006. "Silymarin Protects against Acute Ethanol-Induced Hepatotoxicity in Mice." *Alcoholism: Clinical and Experimental Research* 30 (3):407–13.

SPI: The Plastics Industry Trade Association. 2009. "Plastics and Health." www .plasticsindustry.org/AboutPlastics/content.cfm?ItemNumber=669&&nav ItemNumber=1126 (accessed August 29, 2011).

Sun, Y., E. M. Hersh, S. L. Lee, M. McLaughlin, T. L. Loo, and G. M. Mavligit. 1983. "Preliminary Observations on the Effects of the Chinese Medicinal Herbs Astragalus Membranaceus and Ligustrum Lucidum on Lymphocyte Blastogenic Responses." *Journal of Biological Response Modifiers* 2 (3):227–37.

Sutton, R. 2008. "EWG Research: Teen Girls' Body Burden of Hormone-Altering Cosmetics Chemicals—Adolescent Exposures to Cosmetic Chemicals of Concern." September. Washington, DC: Environmental Working Group. www.ewg.org/reports/teens (accessed April 21, 2011).

Szabo, L. 2009. "Radiation from CT Scans Linked to Cancers, Deaths." *USA Today*, December 14. http.usatoday.com/news/health/2009-12-15-radiation15 _st_N.htm (accessed October 15, 2010).

Takahashi, O., and S. Oishi. 2000. "Disposition of Orally Administered 2,2-Bis(4-Hydroxyphenyl)propane (Bisphenol A) in Pregnant Rats and the Placental Transfer to Fetuses." *Environmental Health Perspectives* 108 (10):931–35.

Tempfer, C. B., E. K. Bentz, S. Leodolter, G. Tscherne, F. Reuss, H. S. Cross, and J. C. Huber. 2007. "Phytoestrogens in Clinical Practice: A Review of the Literature." *Fertility and Sterility* 87 (6):1243–49.

Thangapazham, R. L., A. K. Singh, A. Sharma, J. Warren, J. P. Gaddipati, and R. K. Maheshwari. 2007. "Green Tea Polyphenols and Its Constituent Epigallocatechin Gallate Inhibits Proliferation of Human Breast Cancer Cells in Vitro and in Vivo." *Cancer Letters* 245 (1–2):232–41.

Thomas, T. 2002. "Benchmarks: Garlic and Cancer Prevention." National Cancer Institute (NCI), benchmarks.cancer.gov/2002/11/garlic-and-cancer -prevention/ (accessed November 5, 2010).

Thompson, L. U., J. M. Chen, T. Li, K. Strasser-Weippl, and P. E. Goss. 2005. "Dietary Flaxseed Alters Tumor Biological Markers in Postmenopausal Breast Cancer." *Clinical Cancer Research* 11 (10):3828–35. doi:10.1158/1078-0432 .CCR-04-2326.

U.S. Environmental Protection Agency (EPA). 2005. "Drinking Water Infrastructure Needs Survey and Assessment." Third Report to Congress, June. EPA 816-R-05-001.

U.S. Preventive Services Task Force (USPSTF). 2009. "Screening for Breast Cancer." www.uspreventiveservicestaskforce.org/uspstf/uspsbrca.htm (accessed January 6, 2011).

Vanchieri, C. 2000. "Cutting Copper Curbs Angiogenesis, Studies Show." *Journal of the National Cancer Institute* 92 (15):1202–03.

Vasudevan, N., S. Ogawa, and D. Pfaff. 2002. "Estrogen and Thyroid Hormone Receptor Interactions: Physiological Flexibility by Molecular Specificity." *Physiological Reviews* 82 (4):923–44. doi:10.1152/physrev.00014.2002.

Vega-Riveroll, L., P. Mondragón, J. Rojas-Aguirre, J. Romero-Romo, G. Delgado, and C. Aceves. 2008. "The Antineoplasic Effect of Molecular Iodine on Human Mammary Cancer Involves the Activation of Apoptotic Pathways and the Inhibition of Angiogenesis." Presentation at San Antonio Breast Cancer Symposium, December 12, Texas.

Verreault, R., J. Brisson, L. Deschênes, and F. Naud. 1989. "Body Weight and Prognostic Indicators in Breast Cancer: Modifying Effect of Estrogen Receptors." *American Journal of Epidemiology* 129 (2):260–68.

von Känel, R., P. J. Mills, and J. E. Dimsdale. 2001. "Short-Term Hyperglycemia Induces Lymphopenia and Lymphocyte Subset Redistribution." *Life Sciences* 69 (3):255–62.

Wallace, J. 2010. "Individualizing Nutrition Protocols to Complement Cancer Care." Presentation at 17th International Symposium on Functional Medicine, May 22, Carlsbad, CA.

Walsh, B. 2009. "Getting Real about the High Price of Cheap Food." *Time*, August 21, www.time.com/time/health/article/0,8599,1917458,00.html#ixzz1JjErHwu8 (accessed April 16, 2011).

Warburg, O. 1966. "The Prime Cause and Prevention of Cancer." Lecture presented to Nobel laureates, June 30, at Lindau, Lake Constance, Germany. Rev. English ed. by Dean Burk, National Cancer Institute, Bethesda, MD. 2nd rev. ed. by Konrad Triltsch, Würzburg, Germany, 1969. As quoted in *Beyond the Curtain: Lifting the Illusions of Perception*, http://beyondthecurtain.wordpress.com/2010/02/22/the-prime-cause-and-prevention-of-cancer-revised-by-dr-otto-warburg/ (accessed August 29, 2011).

Way, T.-D., M.-C. Kao, and J. K. Lin. 2004. "Apigenin Induces Apoptosis through Proteasomal Degradation of HER2/*neu* in HER2/*neu*-Overexpressing Breast Cancer Cells via the Phosphatidylinositol 3-Kinase/Akt-dependent Pathway." *Journal of Biological Chemistry* 279 (6):4479–89. doi:10.1074/jbc.M305529200.

World Health Organization (WHO) International Agency for Research on Cancer (IARC). 2006. "Preamble to the IARC Monographs: Scientific Review and Evaluation—Studies of Cancer in Experimental Animals." Lyon,

France: WHO IARC. monographs.iarc.fr/ENG/Preamble/currentb3studies animals0706.php (accessed October 7, 2010).

Wright, J. V. 2005. "Bio-Identical Steroid Hormone Replacement: Selected Observations from 23 Years of Clinical and Laboratory Practice." *Annals of the New York Academy of Sciences* 1057:506–24.

Wright, J. V., and L. Lenard. 2010. *Stay Young and Sexy with Bio-Identical Hormone Replacement: The Science Explained.* Petaluma, CA: Smart Publications.

Yager, J. D., and N. E. Davidson. 2006. "Estrogen Carcinogenesis in Breast Cancer." *New England Journal of Medicine* 354:270–82.

Yahara, T., T. Koga, S. Yoshida, S. Nakagawa, H. Deguchi, and K. Shirouzu. 2003. "Relationship between Microvessel Density and Thermographic Hot Areas in Breast Cancer." *Surgery Today* 33 (4):243–48. doi:10.1007/s005950300055.

Yamasaki-Miyamoto, Y., M. Yamasaki, H. Tachibana, and K. Yamada. 2009. "Fucoidan Induces Apoptosis through Activation of Caspase-8 on Human Breast Cancer MCF-7 Cells." *Journal of Agricultural and Food Chemistry* 57 (18):8677–82. doi:10.1021/jf9010406.

Yance Jr., D. R. 1999. *Herbal Medicine, Healing, and Cancer: A Comprehensive Program for Prevention and Treatment.* With A. Valentine. Chicago: Keats Publishing.

Yi, W., Y., J. Fischer, G. Krewer, and C. C. Akoh. 2005. "Phenolic Compounds from Blueberries Can Inhibit Colon Cancer Cell Proliferation and Induce Apoptosis." *Journal of Agricultural and Food Chemistry* 53 (18):7320–29. doi:10.1021/jf051333o.

Zhang, M., J. Huang, X. Xie, and C. D. Holman. 2009. "Dietary Intakes of Mushrooms and Green Tea Combine to Reduce the Risk of Breast Cancer in Chinese Women." *International Journal of Cancer* 124 (6):1404–08.

Zhang, S., D. J. Hunter, M. R. Forman, B. A. Rosner, F. E. Speizer, G. A. Colditz, J. E. Manson, S. E. Hankinson, and W. C. Willett. 1999. "Dietary Carotenoids and Vitamins A, C, and E and Risk of Breast Cancer." *Journal of the National Cancer Institute* 91 (6):547–56.

Zhang, S. M., W. C. Willett, J. Selhub, J. E. Manson, G. A. Colditz, and S. E. Hankinson. 2003. "A Prospective Study of Plasma Total Cysteine and Risk of Breast Cancer." Cancer Epidemiology, Biomarkers, and Prevention 12 (11, pt. 1):1188–93.

Zowczak, M., M. Iskra, L. Torliński, and S. Cofta. 2001. "Analysis of Serum Copper and Zinc Concentrations in Cancer Patients." *Biological Trace Element Research* 82 (1–3):1–8. doi:10.1385/BTER:82:1-3:001.

**Edward Bauman, MEd, PhD,** is the president and founder of Bauman College: Holistic Nutrition and Culinary Arts. He is a groundbreaking leader in the fields of whole-food nutrition, holistic health, and community health promotion, working to bring his *Eating for Health* approach to schools, community organizations and clinical health care settings. Bauman College has campus locations in Berkeley, CA; Santa Cruz, CA; Penngrove, CA; and Boulder, CO, and also has a distance learning program.

**Helayne Waldman, MS, EdD,** is a holistic nutrition educator with a passion for empowering those with breast cancer. A faculty member at Bauman College: Holistic Nutrition and Culinary Arts, Waldman is a columnist, private practitioner, and consultant to breast cancer clinics and doctors in the San Francisco Bay Area.

Foreword writer **Donald I. Abrams, MD,** is professor of clinical medicine at the University of California, San Francisco, and chief of hematology/oncology at San Francisco General Hospital. He provides integrative oncology consultations at the UCSF Osher Center for Integrative Medicine.

# INDEX

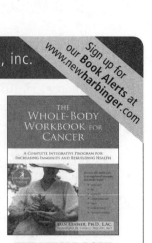
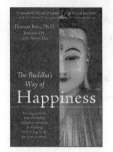
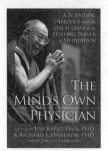
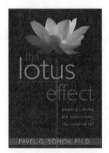
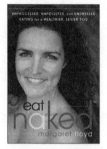
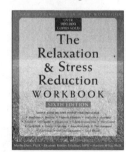
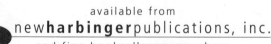